WILDERNESS MEDICAL SOCIETY

Practice Guidelines
for Wilderness
Emergency Care

Edited by

William W. Forgey, M.D.

with 30 contributors

also including the:

Wilderness Pre-hospital Emergency Care Curriculum
suggested by the Wilderness Medical Society for inclusion in the
instruction of Wilderness Emergency Medical Technicians (EMT-W).

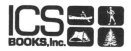

ICS BOOKS, Inc.
Merrillville, Indiana

WILDERNESS MEDICAL SOCIETY PRACTICE GUIDELINES FOR WILDERNESS EMERGENCY CARE

Copyright © 1995 Wilderness Medical Society
Cover photo copyright © 1995 Ken Zafren, M.D.
10 9 8 7 6 5 4 3 2 1

Printed in the U.S.A.

recycled paper

All ICS titles are printed on 50% recycled paper from pre-consumer waste. All sheets are processed without using acid.

Published by:
ICS BOOKS, Inc.
1370 E. 86th Place
Merrillville, IN 46410
800-541-7323

LIBRARY OF CONGRESS CATALOGING-IN-PUBLICATION DATA

Wilderness Medical Society.
    Wilderness Medical Society practice guidelines for wilderness emergency care / edited by Wm. W. Forgey.
        p.   cm.
    Includes index.
    ISBN 1-57034-011-0
    1. Mountaineering injuries. 2. First aid in illness and injury. 3. Wilderness survival.
4. Medical emergencies. I. Forgey, William W., 1942 -   . II. Title.
    [DNLM: 1. Emergencies. 2. Wounds and Injuries--therapy. 3. Travel.
4. Recreation.   WB 105 W673w 1994]
RC88.9.M6W54   1994
616.02'5--dc20
DNLM/DLC
for Library of Congress   94-41746
                                                                            CIP

Table of Contents

Foreword

The last edition of the position papers of the Wilderness Medical Society was issued in 1989. This version, now more appropriately called "practice guidelines," has expanded the topics from 15 to 23.

The previous edition discussed "levels of care," listing different appropriate responses by the lay public, paramedics, and advanced providers. This has been eliminated. The society feels that there is an appropriate response to the various subjects selected, and that this response should be taught to anyone potentially responsible for backcountry medical care. This concept takes us the next logical step beyond standard urban first aid to a new first aid, a wilderness first aid.

Many of the members of the Wilderness Medical Society have been advocating this advance to a more appropriate method of approaching the problems of remote area care for a long time, some long before the society was founded. The WMS has provided the forum to bring the researchers together with the real users of this information, to meld ivy tower concepts with the realities of the field. It has encouraged the formation of a cadre of experts who have been able to glean their knowledge from their interactions within the society.

To further utilize these experts and to assist in the dissemination of this information to the public at large, the society has established a Regional Lay Program Committee. Through this vehicle, members of the society will be establishing workshops across the country elaborating on portions of these practice guidelines. Persons interested in attending one of these meetings are encouraged to contact the society office, or me, for information concerning a program in their area.

The back of this book also lists the annual and specialty meetings of the society. Our meetings provide continuing medical education credit for attending professionals. While they are structured for a physician audience, most lectures and hand-on workshops would be of value to anyone with a background in emergency care or search and rescue. If you have a strong interest in wilderness medicine, you are urged to attend. Please contact the society office for registration materials.

I wish to personally thank the 30 other contributors who participated in either the original set of papers or this updated version. I particularly wish to thank the society president, Warren Bowman, M.D., the members of the Publication Committee (Paul Auerbach, M.D., and William Robinson, M.D.) and the Board of Directors (Howard Backer, M.D., Edward Geehr, M.D., Edward Otten, M.D.*, Bruce Paton, M.D., Douglas Gentile, M.D., Susan Snider, M.D., Ken Zafren, M.D.*, James, Bagian, M.D., Lily Conrad, M.D., Robert Schoene, M.D., and Eric Weiss, M.D.*), some of whom spent considerable energy in multiple reviews and rewrites of these guidelines.

I particularly esteem the efforts of certain associate members of the society for their work during multiple reviews of these papers. To have a dynamic involvement in this project by many of the persons who are actively practicing and teaching wilderness medicine in the field has been invaluable. To this regard I direct my special appreciation to Melissa Grey, Tod Schimelpfenig, and Buck Tilton.

William W. Forgey, M.D.
Editor, Practice Guidelines
Regional Program Chair
Board Member, WMS

812 North West Street
Crown Point, IN 46307

*Also denotes membership on the Publications Committee.

Introduction

"Wilderness," wrote E. O. Wilson, eminent Harvard professor, "settles peace on the soul because it needs no help; it is beyond human contrivance. Wilderness is a metaphor for unlimited opportunity."[1]

Many of us can identify with Wilson's expression of personal need and love for wilderness. We also know that in places that lie geographically far from definitive care, medical problems may arise that many of us are not trained to deal with appropriately. These Position Papers of the Wilderness Medical Society are merely guidelines; your personal level of training, experience, and expertise will determine your willingness and ability to put into practice what we recommend. If you travel into wilderness (defined as a remote geographical location more than one hour from definitive medical care) with the medical responsibility for a group, we recommend - on a moral, ethical and legal basis - that you acquire the needed training, experience, and expertise before going.

The Society has made every effort to ensure the accuracy and appropriateness of these recommendations. References to specific products are incorporated as part of the guidelines, and they are not intended to be endorsements by WMS.

The Wilderness Medical Society wishes to thank members who contributed, some of them many long hours, to these Position Statements:

Howard Backer, M.D.

Richard Banta, M.D.

Warren Bowman, M.D.

Keith Conover, M.D.

Richard Dart, M.D.

Fred Darvill, Jr., M.D.

Steve Donelan

Blair Erb, M.D.

John A. Feagin, Jr., M.D.

William Forgey, M.D.

Edward Geehr, M.D.

Paul Gill, Jr., M.D.

J. Richard Gorham, Ph.D.

Philip Goodman, M.D.

Melissa Gray, EMT-I/C

Peter Hackett, M.D.

Kenneth Iserson, M.D.

Linda Lindsey, RN, EMT

Michael Mackan, M.D.

Sherman A. Minton, M.D.

James Mohle, M.D.

Bruce C. Paton, M.D.

Ramon Ryan, M.D.

Tod Schimelpfenig, EMT-I/C

Joseph Serra, M.D.

Jay Skidmore, Ph.D.

Daniel Spaite, M.D.

John Sullivan, M.D.

Buck Tilton, M.S., EMT-W

Eric A. Weiss, M.D.

Ken Zafren, M.D.

[1] Wilson, E. O.: *The Diversity of Life*, Harvard University Press, Cambridge, 1992.

CHAPTER ONE

Wilderness Evacuation

■ I. GENERAL INFORMATION:

The mode and urgency of the evacuation should be appropriate for the problem. Calling for on-site evacuation, e.g. helicopter, versus leading the victim to care by foot or on a litter, must be decided upon in view of multiple factors including: 1) severity of the illness or injury, 2) rescue and medical skill of the rescuers, 3) physical/psychological condition of the rescuers and/or victims, including the motivation of the group to care for the patient and possibly alter trip plans, timetables and goals, 4) availability of equipment and/or aid for the rescue, 5) the danger/difficulty of extracting the victim(s) by the various means available, 6) time, a product of distance, terrain, weather, and multiple other variables, and 7) cost.

Party leaders must know the capabilities of rescue organizations in the area the group is using and how to contact those organizations. All wilderness leaders must leave trip plans with a responsible person who can act in the group's behalf. If rescue by an outside group (rather than self-rescue by the party) has been determined to be the best course of action, the earlier it is initiated the better. Waiting may allow deterioration of the weather or the patient, and may jeopardize the entire rescue operation.

When requesting outside assistance, the safety of in-comingrescuers, their time commitment, and the cost of the rescue must be considered. It is important to note that the safety of the rescuers or the group takes precedence over ideal management of the patient. Optimally, evacuation decisions must be made by the entire group, including the patient. The potential ecological damage that can occur to the wilderness rescue site from large numbers of rescuers entering the area would argue in favor of a self rescue, if possible.

In general, it is appropriate to postpone further travel and/or initiate evacuation from the wilderness for any person who has the following:

1. Sustained or progressive physiological deterioration, manifested by orthostatic dizziness, syncope, tachycardia, bradycardia, dyspnea, altered mental status, progressive weakness, or intractable vomiting and/or diarrhea, inability to tolerate oral fluids, or the return of loss of consciousness following head injury. In other words, if patients are not improving, they must get out!

2. Debilitating pain.

3. Inability to sustain travel at a reasonable pace due to a medical problem.

4. Passage of blood by mouth or per rectum, if not from an obviously minor source.

5. Signs and symptoms of serious high altitude illness.

6. Infections that progress despite the administration of appropriate treatment.

7. Chest pain that is not clearly musculoskeletal in origin.

8. The development of a dysfunctional psychological status that impairs the safety of the person or the group.

Travel may continue if it is towards definitive care in the case of points 3, 4, and 8, or when descending in the case of point 5 above.

■ II. GUIDELINES FOR GROUND EVACUATION

If the decision has been made for a member of the party to walk out to obtain definitive care, the individual must not go alone. Whenever possible, at least two members of the party, who are mentally and physically equipped to do so, must accompany the patient.

If anything more complex than a simple walk-out of the patient is required, e.g. a litter carry, an on-site leader must be identified who will assume responsibility for the evacuation. If an outside rescue is to be requested, a decision must be made on the most efficacious method of requesting this help. This will often require detaching one, preferably two, members of the party to notify authorities that assistance is needed. This request must be carried in writing and include an assessment of the patient, of the situation to include equipment, personnel, food, water, and a detailed location (map preferred) of the patient. Experience shows that taking the time to write out a detailed note actually decreases total evacuation time. In assessing the anticipated length of evacuation time, the note must include the expertise and rescue experience of the persons in the field with the victim. In many countries a method of payment must be indicated before a rescue will be made.

During a litter evacuation, at least four, and preferably six, bearers must handle the litter at all times. Additional personnel must be available to relieve those handling the litter. The number of litter carriers will ideally be 8 per 100 meters over rough terrain and 6 per 100 meters over reasonably smooth trail. It is very demanding to carry a loaded litter for more than 15 to 20 minutes without a significant break. Litter-carries, especially over rugged terrain, can be agonizingly slow. One bearer will be in charge of the litter, directing lifting and moving, directing the passing of the litter over obstacles, and assuming responsibility for continuously monitoring and reassuring the patient. Many teams standardize the position at the left front of the litter as the litter "driver's" position.

The patient must be carefully "packaged" in the litter for maximum safety and comfort. Protect the patient's head and eyes. Pad stress points, e.g. where the straps press against the body, and the voids, e.g. in the small of the back and behind the knees. Protect from wind, cold, and precipitation. To prevent decubitus ulcers, have the patient move occasionally or alter the patient's position at least every two hours if unconscious. Expect to handle urine and fecal elimination by allowing the functional patient to leave the stretcher with assistance (if serious spine injuries can be cleared), or provide appropriate tilting and/or cleansing toweling to catch excrement. To prevent deep vein thrombosis it is necessary to allow leg movement, or to move or massage legs hourly, as long as this does not increase the trauma of the original injury. If the litter is improvised, test the system and padding first on an uninjured person.

■ III. GUIDELINES FOR HELICOPTER EVACUATION

Helicopters can significantly reduce the time to definitive care when used for emergency transportation of the sick or injured. The decision to use a helicopter for an evacuation must take into account clinical, logistical, and environmental factors. Using a helicopter always adds an element of risk both to rescuers and victim. This risk must be balanced against the risk to the patient, other members of the party, or the rescue team if the patient is evacuated by ground. Evacuate by helicopter only if: 1) a victim's life will be saved, 2) the victim has a significantly better chance for full recovery via a helicopter evacuation, 3) the pilot believes that conditions are safe enough to do the evacuation, 4) a ground evacuation may be unusually dangerous to the ground crew, 5) ground evacuation would be excessively prolonged, or 6) there are not enough rescuers available for a ground evacuation.

Three important points must be kept in mind: 1) evacuating a patient by ground may be faster than waiting for a helicopter (especially in high risk flight conditions); 2) begin evacuation by ground if the helicopter may not be able to respond, or some removal from the accident site would benefit the patient, e.g. descent for altitude sickness; 3) patient may need to be moved to an appropriate landing site; and 4) do not use a helicopter to recover a corpse under emergency conditions.

A. Aircraft Limitations

Helicopters have various configurations, with different capabilities, and different crew skill levels. All helicopters are adversely affected by increased altitude, high environmental temperature, high wind, and heavy payload. The aircraft pilot makes the ultimate decisions concerning flight operations. A helicopter must not fly into known icing conditions or into even moderate storm conditions. Winds over 45 mph, night flights into mountains, and landing in high winds are extremely hazardous. Not all helicopters or pilots are capable of flying by instruments into cloudy or foggy conditions. Party leaders must be familiar with ground-to-air signals, and if radio communication is available, the ground crew must keep the helicopter crew updated on weather and other related conditions at the scene.

Landing and taking off are the two most dangerous activities for both the air and ground crews. As altitude increases, the ability to make vertical hovers and land in small areas is greatly reduced. The optimal landing zone (LZ) is large, well-marked, relatively flat with a slope dropping slightly away from the LZ, and has no tall objects on the perimeter, and no loose debris that could be thrown up by the rapidly spinning blades. The LZ may have to be prepared by the on-site personnel. It must be far enough from the patient so any maneuvering by the helicopter does not put the patient at risk.

The on-site personnel handling the patient must have some familiarity with helicopter operations. Wind generated by the helicopter is tremendous, and all ground personnel must protect themselves when the aircraft lands and takes off. In winter the wind chill from the rotor blades can cause frostbite. Never approach a helicopter until a signal has been given by one of the aircraft personnel. Never approach a helicopter from the rear where the fast–spinning tail rotor is invisible and therefore dangerous, unless it is a rear-entry aircraft and the safe-approach signal has been clearly understood. Once on the ground, all directions from the aircraft crew must be followed explicitly.

B. Aeromedical Considerations

The mechanics and physiology of flight must be understood if it is to be safely used for patient transport. Noise and vibration levels are high, and it may be difficult to monitor, or even communicate with, the patient in flight without special equipment. Helicopter cabins are not pressurized. Atmospheric and oxygen pressure go down as the aircraft goes up. Supplemental oxygen must be available for all patients. Medical devices with air bladders, e.g. MAST, air splints, endotracheal tubes, must be monitored for over–inflation. Ground transport may be a safer alternative for patients with a suspected pneumothorax, decompression sickness, or air embolism.

■ IV. CONTROVERSIES:

A. Is it appropriate to request aided evacuation from the wilderness? Evacuations from the wilderness create risk for the rescuers and are very expensive. In this country, it is assumed that a cry for help will bring an immediate response, free of charge. Especially in less developed countries, it is not always ethical to call for assistance since many native peoples require but cannot afford a life-saving evacuation. Groups traveling into wilderness regions must be able to evacuate themselves. Request assistance as a last resort.

B. Should helicopters be utilized in wilderness areas? Wilderness, by definition, is a place where humans and their conveniences are a transient phenomenon, leaving little or no sign of their passing. Helicopters are an intrusion into wilderness, and the implications of non-essential use of helicopters in wilderness areas is an ethical issue.

CHAPTER TWO

Cardiopulmonary Resuscitation

■ I. GENERAL INFORMATION

Guidelines for the general use of cardiopulmonary resuscitation (CPR) are well-defined, regularly updated, and widely distributed. Because the wilderness may impose circumstances that require special considerations in CPR, the following guidelines have been developed.

A. Contraindications to CPR in the Wilderness

There is no reason to initiate CPR if there is: 1) any sign of life in the patient (pulse, breathing, movement, heart sounds, or recognizable rhythm on a monitor); 2) danger to rescuers; 3) dependent lividity; 4) rigor mortis; 5) obvious lethal injury, e.g. decapitation; 6) a well-defined Do Not Resuscitate (DNR) status; or 7) a patient with a rigid frozen chest. Criteria 3 and 4 may be difficult to evaluate in the non–frozen, yet profoundly hypothermic person (see below) and without documentation criteria 6 is impossible to determine.

B. Discontinuation of CPR in the Wilderness

Once initiated, CPR must be continued until: 1) resuscitation is successful; 2) rescuers are exhausted; 3) rescuers are placed in danger; 4) patient is turned over to more definitive care; or 5) patient does not respond to resuscitative efforts, (see Specific Situations).

C. Rescue Breathing

Initiate rescue breathing if respirations are very shallow or very slow.

■ II. SPECIFIC SITUATIONS

A. Hypothermia:

A cold, rigid, apparently pulseless and breathless patient is not necessarily a dead patient. If you fail to find respiration, initiate rescue breathing immediately. The patient needs oxygen, and there is no danger to the patient from rescue breathing. A cold patient with no detectable pulse should not necessarily be given chest compressions. Apparent lack of pulse may be caused by hypothermia and the resulting tissue rigidity in combination with a very slow heart rate. Chest compressions may trigger ventricular fibrillation, and will not be effective in someone dead from the cold. Do not initiate chest compressions in a patient with a rigid, frozen chest. Rescue breathing, preferably with supplemental oxygen, and immediate gentle evacuation are indicated. Do not use intermittent chest compressions as this technique may induce ventricular fibrillation, further compromising the circulation. If it is decided to initiate chest compressions, this technique must be continued by rescuers without interruption until the victim arrives at the Emergency Department.

B. Avalanche Victims:
Breathless and pulseless victims of avalanches are usually dead from suffocation and/or blunt trauma. Hypothermia is often a confounding factor. Clear the airway, protect the cervical spine, and initiate rescue breathing and chest compressions (CPR) immediately. If there is no response, consider stopping compressions as there has never been a successful resuscitation in a blunt trauma/arrest avalanche victim. Assess and treat concurrent trauma as necessary.

C. Cold-Water Submersion:
Near-drowning patients have occasionally been successfully resuscitated after prolonged (over 1 hour) submersion in cold water (5 to 10° C). Successful resuscitation and favorable outcome are associated with young age, clean water, cold water, short duration of immersion, and pulse present or returning on scene with rescue breathing. Immediately initiate chest compressions and rescue breathing (CPR) and continue, if possible, until definitive care is available.

D. Lightning Strike
Initiate rescue breathing and chest compressions (CPR) immediately on all pulseless, breathless victims of lightning strike. Following a severe electrical shock, respiratory paralysis may persist long after cardiac activity returns. Rescuers must be prepared to provide prolonged resuscitation. If there are multiple victims, reverse normal triage principles, i.e. treat seemingly dead victims first.

CHAPTER THREE

Near Drowning

■ I. GENERAL INFORMATION

Rescue of a drowning victim is inherently dangerous. The following guidelines are suggested for getting the victim safely out of the water: 1) **Reach** for the victim, if possible, with an extended arm or leg, clothing, a stick or paddle, or anything that allows the rescuer to stay safely on land or in a boat. 2) When reaching is not possible, **throw** something that floats to the victim. 3) Throw a line to the victim and **tow** the victim to safety. 4) **Row** or paddle out to drowning victims, in a boat, wearing a personal flotation device. 5) If all else fails, **go** to the victim in a swimming rescue. Swimming rescues are extremely dangerous and are not recommended unless the rescuer has been trained and understands the risk involved.

■ II. GUIDELINES FOR ASSESSMENT AND TREATMENT

Assess unconscious patients immediately for adequate respiration. This can sometimes be done in the water, if the rescuer is a strong swimmer and/or if the rescuer can stand in shallow water. Begin rescue breathing as soon as possible. There is no value in attempting to clear the patient's lungs of water, but be prepared to roll the patient and clear the airway should water fill the airway during the rescue, or if the patient vomits. Performing the Heimlich maneuver on a near–drowned victim is not recommended unless it is impossible to ventilate the patient. It is then done to relieve an obstructed airway only if a finger sweep is not successful. Protect the spine in unconscious patients and in diving or surfing accidents. In the absence of a pulse, begin chest compressions as soon as possible. Evaluate all patients for predisposing factors such as hypoglycemia, seizure and trauma, and from resultant hypothermia who respond to treatment and all near-drowning patients who may have aspirated water and evacuate them to definitive medical care as soon as possible. Even if the victim feels "ok," it is possible to develop delayed respiratory, renal, or other problems, so that evacuation is still indicated. Remember: immediate treatment primarily by ventilation at the scene is the most important factor in determining survival.

CHAPTER FOUR

Head Injury

■ I. GENERAL INFORMATION

Anyone with a blow to the head or face, whether blunt or penetrating, risks developing increased intracranial pressure (ICP) or intracranial bleeding (ICB). Because definitive management of increasing ICP or ICB is not possible in the wilderness, prevent head injuries. Prevention involves attention to safety and includes wearing an adequate helmet, approved for the specific activity being undertaken. It must fit the user and be held in place with a non–stretching chin strap. The use of even a properly fitted helmet does not preclude the risk of ICP if a head injury is sustained, but it can significantly decrease the likelihood. Chin straps should not obstruct venous blood flow as this may cause ICP.

■ II. GUIDELINES FOR ASSESSMENT

Some individuals after a blow to the head or face are low-risk and not in need of immediate evacuation. These patients have had a relatively trivial injury, do not lose consciousness or lose consciousness for less than thirty seconds before returning to a full normal alertness, and have no history of a bleeding disorder or the use of medications which might increase the risk of bleeding. Monitor patients in this category for 24 hours and awaken every 2 hours for assessment. Watch for: 1)alterations in mental status, including personality changes, lethargy, drowsiness, disorientation, unusual irritability, and combativeness; 2) persistent nausea and vomiting; 3) loss of visual acuity; and 4) alterations in coordination and/or speech. If these signs or symptoms of increasing ICP or ICB appear, then an evacuation should be initiated.

Immediate evacuation is recommended for all patients who have received a blow to the head or face that results in loss of consciousness for more than 2 minutes or who have significant signs or symptoms of ICB, increasing ICP, or a depressed or basilar skull fracture. These signs and symptoms include 1) debilitating headache, 2) alterations in mental status (see above), 3) persistent nausea and vomiting, 4) Battle's sign (ecchymosis behind and below the ears), 5) raccoon eyes (periorbital ecchymosis), 6) loss of coordination, 7) loss of visual acuity, 8) appearance of clear fluid (possibly cerebral spinal fluid) from the nose and/or ears, 9) seizures, and 10) relapse into unconsciousness.

■ III. GUIDELINES FOR TREATMENT

If there is an obvious head injury consider the possibility of a cervical spine injury (see Spinal Injury). Specific measures to implement during evacuation include: Establishing and maintaining an airway in all unconscious patients is of critical importance. Airway management, without specific adjuncts, can usually be accomplished by keeping the patient in a stable side position, which also helps alleviate the possibility of aspirating vomitus, a common threat with head-injured patients. Alternatively, with consideration for possible spinal injury, place patient with his/her head elevated 30° to decrease the chance of aspiration. There is no consensus with regard to the value of hyperventilation in these patients.

While all persons with a mechanism of injury which includes head involvement are strapped to a backboard in an urban setting, this is not necessary if the patient assessment does not indicate that evacuation is required. When evacuation is initiated, reassessment of the requirement for neck or spine immobilization should be made periodically. If the spine can be cleared, the rigid immobilization should be terminated, even through the evacuation process is continued.

CHAPTER FIVE

Spinal Injury

■ I. GENERAL INFORMATION

In an urban environment, many patients placed in full spinal immobilization will prove not to have unstable spine injuries, but the inconvenience to patients and rescuers is worth the extra effort to protect the few who do. The decision to initiate and to maintain cervical spine immobilization in the wilderness has significant ramifications. An otherwise ambulatory patient who could facilitate his or her own evacuation would need an expensive and potentially hazardous rescue. The added delay could exacerbate other injuries and predispose the victim and the rescue party to hypothermia or other environmental hazards.

Immobilize all patients with signs or symptoms as indicated below in "assessment." Patients with no signs or symptoms need not be immobilized despite significant mechanisms of injury, unless they have an altered level of responsiveness.

■ II. GUIDELINES FOR ASSESSMENT AND TREATMENT

In the wilderness a number of steps are involved in ruling out a spinal injury in a patient with a positive mechanism of injury. If the patient fails a step at any point in the process, treatment begins. Treatment consists of full immobilization in a rigid litter, or immobilization on the most level ground available with a cervical collar until a rigid litter can be improvised or brought in.

Treat the patient for spinal injury unless he or she is fully alert. Patients complaining of neck pain (not just "tightness") or altered peripheral sensations should be treated for spinal injury. Test the patient for motor and sensory function in the extremities. Treat for spinal injury if there is any deficit. Gently palpate the patient's spine. Treat the patient if there is marked tenderness, or there is significant spasm or guarding. While supporting the head, have the patient move his or her head slowly through a normal range of motion. Immobilize the patient if movement results in any axial pain. If movement results in no pain, the patient may be allowed to move freely but carefully. If at any point the patient begins to complain of pain, weakness, or numbness, immobilize the spine.

■ III. CONTROVERSIES

Should all patients with a suspected spinal injury be immobilized and evacuated? In the wilderness, full spinal immobilization may pose unnecessary hardship and danger to patients and rescuers. Therefore, seek a balance between the difficulties and dangers of evacuating an immobilized patient on one hand and not immobilizing a spinal injury on the other. In certain hazardous situations, it may be safer for the patient and rescuers to forgo spinal immobilization, or to use only partial spinal immobilization such as a cervical collar alone, to evacuate more easily and rapidly from the area of immediate danger.

CHAPTER SIX

Wilderness Wound Management

■ I. GENERAL INFORMATION

Assume contamination of open wounds and treat accordingly. The major goals are: 1) stop blood loss; 2) clean the wound and keep it clean; 3) promote healing and reduce discomfort; and 4) minimize loss of function. Most wilderness first aid kits contain simple bandages and compresses only. Improvisation and the use of substitute materials are often required.

■ II. GUIDELINES FOR ASSESSMENT AND TREATMENT

Wear fluid barrier gloves when contacting blood or other body fluids, unless unavailable or if a delay would be harmful to the patient. Improvised personal protection could include, for example, a plastic food bag or piece of garment to minimize contact with the victim's blood and sunglasses or ski goggles to protect your eyes.

Even *heavy bleeding* can be controlled with pressure techniques in nearly all instances. Initially, apply direct digital pressure over the bleeding vessels and elevate the wound. Pressure is best applied through a dressing, such as a wad of gauze or clean cloth. A pressure dressing (such as a strip of cloth tied over a wad of gauze) may also control bleeding. Pressure points alone are not effective as a primary technique to control bleeding, but may be useful as an adjunct. Arterial tourniquets are rarely necessary and, if used, they must be released every 5 minutes, while continuing to apply direct wound pressure, to assess the continued need for the tourniquet.

Treat *contusions* during the first 48 hours with cold compresses or cold water immersion, and a compression dressing, to limit expanding hematomas and to aid in pain relief. Apply cold for one half hour every two hours with due regard to possible cold injury. After 72 hours, apply heat in the same manner to promote healing. Topical heat ointments or creams can cause skin irritation, and their use is discouraged. Large contused areas with marked swelling cause severe pain and disability and may signal a large amount of blood loss or a significant underlying injury. Evaluate such patients for shock and other possible injuries and treated accordingly. *Do not drain hematomas.* A major soft tissue injury in proximity to a bone should arouse a high suspicion of a fracture. Apply splints for comfort.

Subungual hematomas may be drained by drilling a hole in the nail with a hot paper clip, a sharp blade, or hypodermic needle to provide pain relief.

Scrub *abrasions* clean with soap and water or with a surgical scrub such as .5% chlorhexidine gluconate or a 1% povidone-iodine impregnated sponge. Follow scrubbing with copious irrigation with the cleanest water available. After the abrasion has been cleaned, apply a thin coating of a topical antimicrobial first-aid ointment and dress with a sterile gauze.

Lacerations and *avulsions* are best cleaned by copious high pressure irrigation using the cleanest water available. Pressure irrigation with a syringe and 18 or 19 gauge needle or catheter is the most effective technique. The ideal irrigation method should produce enough pressure to dislodge bacteria and debris without causing tissue damage. Improvised equipment could include a plastic bag with a small hole in it. This method is less effective than the syringe and catheter system, however, because it fails to generate adequate pressure.

Use of non-disinfected water is discouraged, unless the wound is grossly contaminated and no other irrigation is available. If using surface water for deep or large wounds, sterilize the water with a ten minute boil or filtration to remove bacterial spores. Boiled then cooled water is safest for open fractures or lacerations over joints. The liquid used to irrigate the wound should be clean and non-toxic to tissues. Sterile normal saline, 1% povidone-iodine and disinfected water are ideal solutions. Stronger disinfectant solutions have no proven benefit over sterile normal saline. Normal saline can be improvised in the backcountry by adding 9 grams of salt (roughly 2 teaspoons) to one liter of disinfected water.

Take care to avoid splashing fluid into the irrigator's face. Following irrigation, inspect the wound and remove remaining debris with a sterile (flamed or boiled) forceps.

Closing contaminated or high risk wounds increases the chance of wound infection. Pack contaminated wounds open if they cannot be thoroughly irrigated. Minor wounds do not require urgent evacuation and may be closed with tape or wound closure strips. Significant wounds are best cleaned and dressed without closure and the patient evacuated for definitive care. If evacuation is not feasible, or will take longer than two days, it is reasonable to treat significant wounds with thorough cleaning and closure with tape, wound closure strips, sutures, or surgical staples. When wound closure is elected, the most sterile environment possible must be created. Limit sharp debridement to obviously devitalized tissue. Splinting and elevation will help maintain wound closure, hemostasis, and pain control.

If bone is exposed or if the wound is a deep puncture or highly contaminated, give appropriate antibiotics. Ascertain tetanus status and give recommendations for updating after leaving the wilderness. Observe wounds daily for signs of infection, indicating the need for further irrigation, drainage, or debridement.

Traumatic amputations necessitate proper management of the amputated body part, if there will be any opportunity for re-implantation. Gently clean the body part and wrap in slightly moist sterile gauze, seal in plastic, and keep as cool as possible without freezing (ice water is best). Some body parts, such as fingers, may be reattached up to 32 hours after the injury.

Vigorously irrigate *animal bites* with the cleanest water available. Except where necessary to control hemorrhage or to allow extrication, never close or tightly approximate an animal bite wound. Give amoxicillin-clavulanate, a 2nd or 3rd generation cephalosporin, a quinolone, a penicillinase resistant penicillin, or a tetracycline antibiotic (erythromycin is not an acceptable alternative).

Consider rabies in bites if: 1) the attack was unprovoked (a bite is not considered provoked if there was any attempt to feed, pet, run by, or capture the animal); 2) the animal was acting unnaturally prior to the bite; 3) the animal is a member of a high-risk species (bats, raccoons, skunks, the canines, and the felines); or 4) the geographic region is a known rabies-infested area. Animals whose bites have never caused rabies in humans in the United States are livestock (cattle, sheep, horse), rabbit, gerbil, chipmunk, squirrel, rat, and mouse. In case of a suspicious bite, rabies immune globulin must be administrated immediately and simultaneously with the human diploid cell rabies vaccine in non–immunized people. Consider rabies prophylaxis prior to travel in remote regions where rabies is prevalent.

■ III. GUIDELINES FOR EVACUATION

Rapid evacuation from the wilderness is advisable for: 1) severe animal bites or bites from potentially rabid animals; 2) deep or highly contaminated wounds with a high risk of infection; 3) wounds that open to fractures (other than the distal phalanx) or to joint spaces; 4) infected wounds not responding promptly to treatment; and 5) wounds associated with severe blood loss. While not an urgent matter, consider evacuation for wounds that severely limit an individual's ability to participate in the trip and wounds that require closure for cosmetic reasons (such as wounds on the face). Delayed primary closure of facial wounds can be performed in 3 to 5 days if the wound is kept clean with daily packing.

■ IV. CONTROVERSIES:

A. Should wounds be closed in the wilderness? Although sterile techniques are virtually impossible in the wilderness, primary closure with sutures, staples or wound closure strips is recommended for relatively clean wounds. Staples provide a cosmetic result identical to that of interrupted sutures, but not subcuticular sutures. The patient's comfort and ability and willingness to function are increased, and healing time is usually shortened. For ulcerations, abscess cavities, deep puncture wounds, and animal bites, do not close wounds but allow to gradually heal by granulation and eventual re-epithelization. Grossly contaminated wounds, excessively contaminated with soil or feces must be cleaned and observed for 4 to 5 days before closure, if the wilderness trip lasts that long.

B. Should antibiotic prophylaxis be considered for wilderness wounds? The following are general indications for antibiotic prophylaxis: 1) significantly contaminated wounds requiring extensive cleaning and debridement (especially in patients with pre-existing valvular heart disease, prosthetic joints, or immunosuppressed patients), 2) violation of cartilage, joint spaces, tendon, or bone, 3) crush-mechanism wounds with a high potential for devitalization, and 4) mammalian bites. See antibiotic suggestions listed above. For prophylaxis, three to five days of therapy suffice.

CHAPTER SEVEN

Burn Management

■ I. GENERAL INFORMATION

The most likely source of major burn trauma in the outdoors is from flammable fuel used in camp stoves and lanterns. Scalds from hot liquids can also cause extensive burns. Thermal injuries from stoves, carbide lights and lanterns, hot utensils, and campfires are generally not extensive, but stress the importance of prevention.

■ II. GUIDELINES FOR ASSESSMENT AND TREATMENT

Every aspect of burn treatment depends on assessment of the depth and extent of the injury. Although this assessment may be an estimate, it is the basis for deciding how the patient will be treated, and whether evacuation is required, and how urgently.

A. Assessment

(1)Depth: First degree burns involve the epidermis only. The skin color is red to pale and no blister forms. Second degree burns have blisters in addition to the red discoloration of the skin. Third degree burns have a pale or charred skin color and do not have blister formation.

(2)Extent: Use the Rule of Nines, in which each arm represents approximately 9% of a person's total body surface area (TBSA), each leg 18% (the front of the leg 9%, and the back of the leg 9%), the front of the torso represents 18% the back of the trunk18%, the head represents 9%, and the groin 1%. For infants and small children, the head represents a larger percentage (18%) and the legs a smaller percentage (13.5%). For smaller areas, use the Rule of Palmar Surface: the patient's palmar surface equals about 1% TBSA.

(3)Pain: In addition to depth and extent, do not underestimate the assessment value of pain. Adequate control of pain is a treatment goal and indicator of the ability to manage a burn wound while in the wilderness.

B. Initial Care:

(1) *Stop the Burning Process.* The faster the better, within 30 seconds, if possible. Heat can continue to injure tissue for a surprisingly long time. No first aid will be effective until the burning process has stopped. Smother flames, if appropriate, then cool the burn with water, unless the burn is greater than 20% of the TBSA, with due regard to causing hypothermia. Remove clothing and jewelry from the burn area. Do not try to remove anything that has stuck to the wound.

(2) *Manage the ABCs.*

(3) *Assess for Associated Injuries* such as fractures or lacerations and inhalation injury.

(4) *Evaluate the Burn* (depth, extent, pain).

(5) *General Treatment for the Patient:*

a. Stabilize the body temperature. When skin is lost, so is the patient's ability to thermoregulate.

b. Have the patient drink as much fluid as he or she can tolerate without vomiting. Include some salt in the oral fluids, but do not make these solutions stronger than .9%. This is the equivalent of a pinch of salt per 8 ounce glass.

c. Remember: altered consciousness is due to a cause other than the burn.

C. General Treatment of the Burn:

Caring for the wound itself is often the least important aspect of burn care. All burn wounds are sterile for the first 24 to 48 hours. Burn management is aimed primarily at keeping the wound clean and reducing the pain.

a. Gently wash the burn with tepid water and mild soap, if needed, to remove any debris and to clean the skin surface around the burn site. Pat dry. Remove the skin from blisters that have popped open or are hemorrhagic (but do not open blisters unless necessary for function of hands or feet).

b. Dress burns with a thin layer of antibiotic ointment.

c. Cover the burn with Spenco 2nd Skin®, if the burn is small enough, or cover with a thin layer of gauze, or clean, dry clothing. Burns on the face, neck and hands may be left open to the air after applying ointment. Covering wounds reduces pain and evaporative losses, but do not use an occlusive dressing.

d. When evacuation is imminent, do not re-dress or re-examine the injury. If evacuation is prolonged, re-dress once a day. Remove old dressings, re-clean (removing the old ointment), and apply fresh ointment and a clean dry covering. (Note: if stuck, soak off old dressings with clean, tepid water.)

e. Do not pack wounds in ice which are larger than 20% of the body surface area. Do not leave wet coverings on burns for more than two hours at a time to reduce the risk of hypothermia.

f. Elevate burned extremities to minimize swelling. Swelling retards healing and encourages infection. Have the patient gently and regularly move burned areas as much as possible.

g. Ibuprofen is probably the best over-the-counter analgesic for burn pain (including sunburn).

h. If you have no ointment or dressings, leave the burn alone. The burn's surface will dry into a scab-like covering that provides a significant amount of protection.

■ III. GUIDELINES FOR EVACUATION

First degree burns, even extensive ones, rarely require evacuation. The initially severe pain resolves within 24 hours. Second degree burns covering less than 15% TBSA must receive definitive care, but seldom warrant rapid evacuation. Third degree burns need definitive medical care to heal best, but do not usually require rapid evacuation unless they are extensive. Second and third degree burns covering more than 15% TBSA are often a threat to life, requiring rapid evacuation. Any serious burn to the face may have burned the patient's airway, and must be considered for rapid evacuation. Third degree burns of hands, feet or genitals require prompt evacuation.

CHAPTER EIGHT

Orthopedic Injuries

■ I. GENERAL INFORMATION

Sprains, strains, and fractures, especially injuries to lower extremities, are the most common accidents in wilderness settings. The treatment of these injuries may vary, depending upon the expertise and experience of those in the party and the distance from definitive medical help. In remote settings, making the patient as functional as possible is often the overriding concern, thereby facilitating self-rescue and eliminating the need for outside assistance. Remember, the safety of the group takes precedence over optimal treatment of any individual injury.

Managing fractures in remote environments requires common sense, good diagnostic skills, and sensitivity to the needs of the patient and the group. For example, in a severe ankle injury where a fracture is suspected, one would normally immobilize the part and put the patient on crutches with instructions for elevation, ice, and rest from weight bearing. In the wilderness, however, one must weigh other factors: the desire of the patient to ambulate on a suspicious ankle injury, the availability of people to transport the patient, the type of terrain involved in transport, the severity of the environment, distance involved, and the patient's need or desire as well as ability to continue carrying a load. Thus, whereas the best medical judgement precludes weight-bearing, the best decision in a remote environment might be to immobilize the ankle in a splint, or tape the ankle securely as for an athletic event, and allow the patient to hobble along on his or her good ankle using an ice axe, ski pole or wooden stick for balance. This could be the safest and most reasonable decision based on the situation.

■ II. GUIDELINES FOR ASSESSMENT AND TREATMENT – FRACTURES

In the wilderness, without a radiographic picture of the involved bones, assessment of a fracture includes the following questions: 1) Are there obvious signs of a fracture, such as angulations, swelling, bruising, or open wound? (In cold environments, perform the examination, as much as possible, by reaching beneath clothing that is left in place.) 2) Can the patient move the injury or does she/he guard it carefully? 3) Is there discoloration and swelling? 4) How does the injured side compare to the uninjured side? 5) Does the injury feel rigid with spasm of the surrounding muscles? 6) Did the patient feel or hear anything break? 7) What was the mechanism of injury? (High-speed impact causes more fractures than low-speed impact). 8) Is there "point tenderness" when the suspected fracture site is touched? 9) Is there adequate circulation distal to the suspected fracture site? and 10) How willing is the patient to use the injured area?

Splinting may be accomplished with formal splints or improvised with clothing, adhesive or athletic tape, foamlite sleeping pads, ice axes, ski poles, or natural material. The key elements of a splint are adequate padding for comfort and adequate rigidity for safety. The patient is the best source of information on how well splints are working. Peripheral pulses must be monitored before and after all splinting. Check pulses periodically to ensure that the splint wrap is not too tight. It is important to give the patient the responsibility of notifying someone of any changes in sensation or level of pain.

A. Shoulder: Fractures of the shoulder girdle are quite often stable and require nothing more than sling immobilization, cold compresses, if available, and allowance for gentle motion of the forearm and hand. A fracture of the clavicle may be treated with a sling and swathe. The hand and wrist must be accessible for feeling pulses.

B. Upper Arm: The humeral shaft is palpable on the medial side throughout its entire length. Therefore, when fracture is suspected palpate the length of the humerus, beginning either proximal or distal to the patient's area of complaint. In this way, very small, non–displaced fractures may be identified. Ask the patient to extend her or his wrist, digits and thumb to check the radial nerve function and document for future reference. Immobilizing the arm against the body wall is nature's best splint. Humeral fractures can be very adequately padded and immobilized in this manner with a sling and swathe. For comfort leave the elbow free and dependent, allowing gravity to apply gentle traction to the fracture site, which is splinted to the thorax with only the swathe. An unstable or displaced humeral fracture may require a padded splint.

C. Lower Arm: Adequately splint fractures of the elbow, forearm, and wrist, incorporating the joints above and below. If possible, splint the elbow at 80 to 90 degrees of flexion to elevate the forearm and hand and reduce swelling.

The stability provided by a rigid splint is worth the effort, especially in a long and difficult transport. Splint fractures of the distal ulna and radius with the hand placed in the position of function with a rolled up sock, glove, or other soft material tucked into the palm. Then immobilize the hand, wrist, and forearm in a splint. Active exercise of the hand is quite helpful in promoting circulation.

Correct marked angulation. Applying a splint to a badly angulated forearm fracture is difficult and usually unstable. Gentle traction with an assistant applying counter-traction to the upper arm results in an overall improvement with a negligible risk of creating further vascular or neurologic damage. Move slowly and stop if force is required for further movement, or the patient complains of significantly increasing pain.

D. Hand: Fractures of the hand are often associated with dislocations of the proximal or distal interphalangeal joints. Reduce phalangeal fractures and splint in a position of function as indicated above, not in an extended position. *Immediately after injury, these fractures can be reduced with only minimal discomfort.* Hours after the injury, swelling and pain make realignment more difficult. Use of an ice compress and very gentle traction can realign fractures of the hand without significant discomfort. Immobilize the digits in a position of function whenever possible, and use adjacent digits for splinting (the "buddy system"). Place gauze between the buddy-taped fingers to absorb moisture. A suitable hand splint may be made by placing the entire hand in a functional position with a soft roll of material in the palm, and then wrapping the whole with an elastic wrap or roller gauze. Torn strips of clothing can be used for an improvised hand splint.

E. Hip: In fractures of the hip, the typical position of external rotation and shortening of the leg may or may not be present. The fracture may be an impacted femoral neck type or an acetabular fracture. Diagnosis might be difficult. As a general guideline, if a patient has sustained significant trauma and has very painful motion in the region of the hip, plus pain with weight-bearing, carry him or her out on a litter or sled. Do not place suspected fractures of the hip in traction. Secure the leg on the affected side to the uninjured leg for splinting.

F. Pelvis: In suspected fractures of the pelvis, treat for shock due to the massive blood loss often associated with this injury. Because of possible bladder trauma, check for hematuria. Gentle constricting wraps placed around the pelvic region may provide temporary comfort and more stability to the fracture. The patient requires stabilization on a rigid backboard, litter, or sled.

G. Femur: Fractures of the femoral shaft must be treated in traction for many important reasons. The most important is that traction re-establishes normal length and conformity of the musculature and tightens the fascial envelope, which tends to decrease the bleeding that occurs in the thigh. A patient with a femoral shaft fracture can easily lose more than a liter of blood into the thigh and, if the fracture is movable and the thigh unstable, this bleeding can continue. Additionally, fracture fragments may cause further vascular damage.

Traction also relieves pain, stabilizes fracture fragments, prevents converting a closed fracture into an open fracture, and reduces further soft-tissue damage. In a major expedition or an extended trek into remote regions, the expedition physician or paramedical person in charge must plan ahead for the type of traction that will be used if a femoral shaft fracture occurs.Commercial traction devices are available that are lightweight, easy to use, and efficient.

Improvised femoral traction can be satisfactory, but must be practiced prior to the actual event, or at least tried out on an uninjured volunteer first, so that everyone understands and is familiar with the plan. Once a fractured femur has been diagnosed, assign someone to apply manual traction to the extremity (with the patient protected from the environment) until the traction device is in place. A general rule for how much traction to apply is 10% of the patient's body weight or until the pain is relieved. Additional immobilization of the fractured extremity to the uninjured leg with adequate padding can also be helpful. When long transport is anticipated, place padding behind the knee to create 5 to 10% knee flexion. This position is much more comfortable than if the knee is fully extended in traction.

Frequently monitor and document circulation distal to the injury. It is not necessary to remove the boot and sock in most instances and may be inadvisable in cold weather. Traction is usually more comfortable with the boot and sock on, and the dorsalis pedis pulse can usually be palpated by sliding a finger under the sock. A gross determination of sensation and skin warmth can be made by palpation. The patient can relate sensations of numbness or tingling in the toes. A complication of the traction splinting techniques which employ an ankle hitch is tissue necrosis of the ankle or foot. This can be avoided by reassessment, removing the traction splint for periods of time, or using tape skin traction with the boot off instead of an ankle hitch.

H. Knee: Patellar fractures from a fall directly on the knee may be difficult to differentiate from a severe contusion unless there is an obvious deformity. A person with a compound fracture of the patella will be unable to extend the knee. Immobilize a patient with severe knee pain in a cylinder splint that stabilizes the knee, and walk with assistance. Improvise a cane or crutch, if terrain and other factors dictate that this is the best course of action.

I. Lower Leg: Splint tibia and both bone fractures to incorporate the knee and ankle. Many isolated fibula fractures require only an ankle splint and the victim can ambulate with a cane or crutch. Traction splinting is unnecessary. Gently correct angular deformities (see Lower Arm above).

J. Ankle: Fractures of the ankle may be difficult to assess. Early examination and treatment are important. Immobilize adequately, then elevate and apply cold to the injured extremity. A well-wrapped compression dressing is also quite helpful. Ankle fractures may be splinted very well with parkas, foam sleeping pads, or other comparable gear arranged in a "U" shape around the foot and lower leg.

■ III. GUIDELINES FOR ASSESSMENT AND TREATMENT - DISLOCATIONS

It is important to diagnose and reduce a dislocation quickly after it occurs. Discretion must obviously be used in deciding to reduce the dislocation when evacuation to a nearby medical facility can be easily accomplished.

The major advantages of early reduction are: 1) Reduction is easier immediately after the injury, before swelling and muscle spasm have developed; 2) Transport of the patient is easier after reduction; 3) Reduction usually results in dramatic relief of pain; 4) Immobilization of the injured joint is easier to accomplish and more stable after reduction; 5) The safety of the entire party may be jeopardized during the evacuation of a patient with a major joint dislocation; 6) Early reduction reduces the circulatory and neurological risks to the extremity.

Signs helpful in identifying a dislocation include: 1) restriction of motion through the joint's normal range, 2) obvious deformity in comparison with the uninvolved side, 3) crepitus or grating of bone fragments is absent, and 4) often a typical, identifiable posture of the dislocated joint, which the patient will maintain to minimize pain. Obtaining a history of the mechanism of injury is helpful.

Avulsion fractures may accompany dislocations. The alignment of these fractures is usually improved with the reduction of the dislocation. The same is true of vessel or nerve impairment associated with a dislocation. When a major long bone fracture (e.g. femur or humerus) accompanies a dislocation in the same area, the dislocation may not even be diagnosed in view of the more apparent major fracture. In these cases, splinting of the fracture is the main concern. The dislocation, for all practical purposes, is a secondary issue, and usually not amenable to reduction by ordinary means.

A. Shoulder: Anterior-inferior dislocations of the shoulder joint account for over 90% of shoulder dislocations. The mechanism of injury is usually external rotation and abduction. The problem is often recurrent and the patient can identify the dislocation quite readily. The patient will usually stabilize the shoulder in the most comfortable position, but cannot bring the involved extremity across the chest to a position of rest. The upper arm is held away from the body in various positions and cannot be brought into a sling-type position. This differentiates a dislocation from a fracture of the humerus, in which the patient usually splints the upper arm against the chest wall for comfort. Check circulation, motor and sensory function to the hand, and also sensory function along the outer aspect of the shoulder (axillary nerve), and document findings.

Posterior dislocations of the shoulder are not common. In this instance, the upper arm and forearm are held across the anterior chest wall and attempts at externally rotating the upper arm away from the chest are restricted and painful. The diagnosis is often difficult to make.

The best method for reduction of an anterior shoulder dislocation is steady traction with the arm abducted 90°, pulling straight from the body with counter-traction provided in the region of the axilla by an assistant. Muscle relaxation through massage can enhance attempts at relocation and is appropriate. Be sure to pad the axilla and the antecubital region to protect nerve and vascular structures during traction.

A second method is to place the patient prone and let the arm hang down toward the ground with 10 to 15 pounds of weight secured to the hand. This method may be slow and relaxation is critically important, but the muscles will generally fatigue in time, and manual assistance by manipulation of the shoulder is helpful.

After reduction, immobilize the shoulder with sling and swathe.

B. Elbow: Look for obvious deformity when compared to the uninvolved side and restricted flexion and extension of the joint. Most commonly, the olecranon dislocates toward the rear and a bony prominence shows posteriorly.

Apply slow, steady traction to the forearm in a partially flexed position with counter-traction applied to the upper arm by an assistant. The patient's ability to fully flex the elbow is a sign of reduction. The joint may be displaced medially or laterally and may require side pressure for realignment. After reduction, immobilize in a sling and swathe. If reduction is not possible, splint in the position found.

C. Wrist: Dislocations are very difficult to differentiate from a fracture, and often difficult to reduce. Splint immobilization is the treatment of choice (see wrist fracture). Circulation and neurologic function to the hand are usually not compromised, but, if they are, attempt reduction with gentle in-line traction.

D. Fingers: Obvious deformity and limited function are the main diagnostic factors. Reduction of dislocations of middle and distal interphalangeal joints is accomplished by maintaining the digit in partial flexion and pushing the dislocated base of the phalanx back in place while traction is applied to the partially flexed digit.

There are two hand dislocations in which reduction is difficult, if not impossible, by closed means: dislocation of the metacarpophalangeal joint of the index finger and the metacarpophalangeal joint of the thumb. The thumb is sometimes reducible closed, but the index metacarpal rarely is. Make one attempt, then immobilize the joint in a functional position. Do not persist with multiple attempts.

E. Hip: The majority of dislocations are posterior. The hip will be moderately flexed, internally rotated and adducted. Any attempt to extend the hip for splinting or easier transport will be resisted by the patient and is mechanically nearly impossible to accomplish. Anterior dislocation of the hip results in a posture of extension, external rotation and abduction. Again, attempting to extend the hip to a neutral position is very difficult, if not impossible, and is resisted by the patient.

If skill and equipment are available, the use of intramuscular or intravenous muscle relaxants or analgesics greatly facilitate any reduction. This reduction requires two people, ideally, with one applying counter-traction to the pelvis with the patient lying in a supine position on the ground. In the case of a posterior hip dislocation, the involved hip and knee are flexed to 90° with the rescuer straddling the patient and applying traction in an upward direction. If only one person is available to attempt the reduction, the victim can be placed prone over a log, rock, or bench, and the traction applied downward with hip and knee flexed 90°. Once reduced, the injured hip must be immobilized to the uninvolved extremity and the patient transported in a supine position.

F. Patella: Most often, the patella is laterally displaced with the knee held in flexion for comfort. Such an injury is often recurrent and caused by a pivoting type of injury with a partially flexed knee. The patella is not movable and is obviously out of place.

Flex the hip to relax the quadriceps, then apply gentle traction to extend the knee while applying direct pressure to the patella from the lateral side, thus pushing it back into the groove. Often, as the knee is extended, the patella will reduce itself. Immobilize the extremity with a cylinder splint. With the knee extended and immobilized, the patient may be able to walk well enough for self evacuation.

G. Knee: Major ligamentous disruption is the rule in dislocations of the knee. The knee may not be dislocated at the time of exam, but gross instability is the major clue, and vascular impairment is an important risk. Check pulses and motor function in ankle and foot.

Gentle realignment of the joint benefits damaged neurovascular structures. Splint securely, without compromising circulation to the foot. The patient must be carried out.

H. Ankle: Most commonly associated with fractures, the dislocated ankle is obviously deformed and often manifests crepitus. Reduce the deformity as much as possible as necrosis of tight, stretched overlying skin is a danger. Ordinarily, this is not difficult because of the gross instability resulting from associated fractures. Hold the forefoot and allow the remainder of the extremity to act as the counter-traction. Improved alignment of the ankle dislocation results without much additional effort. Gentle traction of the heel and foot also helps. Immobilize with a splint, and carry the patient out.

■ IV. GUIDELINES FOR EVACUATION

Deciding which injuries mandate premature termination of a trip, and how rapidly and by what means evacuation will be performed, is a function of both the type of trip and type of injury. Rapid evacuation is indicated in: 1) open fractures, 2) injuries with vascular compromise not alleviated by reduction, 3) spinal injuries with neurologic deficits, and 4) injuries associated with significant blood loss. Evacuation is not needed for: 1) digit injuries and 2) minimal injuries to other joints. With adequate splinting, delays in reaching definitive medical care often result in no permanent harm.

CHAPTER NINE

High-Altitude Illness

■ I. GENERAL INFORMATION

High-altitude illnesses affect large numbers of wilderness travelers and result in occasional deaths. The most common illnesses are acute mountain sickness (AMS), high-altitude pulmonary edema (HAPE), high altitude cerebral edema (HACE), and peripheral edema. Proper management requires early diagnosis and prompt intervention. In the field, the safety of rescuers or the group may take precedence over ideal management of the patient.

■ II. GUIDELINES FOR PREVENTION

Most altitude illness is preventable. The following measures reduce the incidence and severity of high-altitude illness. Although these measures do not guarantee freedom from illness, they are highly recommended, especially for those without altitude experience.

A. Staged Ascent: Acclimatize by gradually increasing the altitude of overnight camps. If possible, the first camp should be no higher than 8000 feet (2400 meters), with an increase of no more than 1000 to 2000 feet (300 to 600 meters) per night. An alternative approach is to spend two nights at the same altitude for every 2000-foot (600 meter) gain in altitude above 10,000 feet (3,000 meters). If a trip is started at over 9000 feet (2,700 meters), two nights should be spent acclimatizing at that altitude before proceeding higher. Proceed higher during the day and return to a lower elevation to sleep (climb high, sleep low).

B. High-Carbohydrate Diet: A diet of at least 70% carbohydrates reduces symptoms of AMS by about 30%, and can be started one to two days prior to ascent.

C. Appropriate Exercise Level: Until acclimatized, exercise moderately, avoiding excessive dyspnea and fatigue.

D. Hydration: To offset increased fluid losses at high altitudes, stay well-hydrated. Adequate hydration may be judged by the presence of clear and copious urination.

E. Drug Prophylaxis: Several drugs can lessen the symptoms of high-altitude illness. However, their use is not recommended as a routine measure.

    1. Acetazolamide – The indications for acetazolamide prophylaxis are a forced rapid ascent, proceeding to sleeping altitude greater than 9000 feet (2,700 meters) in one day from less than

4000 feet (1,200 meters), or a history of previous AMS at similar rates of ascent. Acetazolamide reduces symptoms of AMS by about 75%. Acetazolamide is considered the drug of choice for chemoprophylaxis of AMS.

The dose of acetazolamide for adults is 125 mg twice a day, starting the day of ascent. The dose for children is 5-10 mg/kg/day, up to the adult dose of 125 mg twice daily.

Common side effects from this drug include peripheral paresthesia and polyuria. Contraindications are pregnancy, metabolic or respiratory acidosis, or allergy to sulfa drugs. Bone marrow suppression occurs, but is rare.

2. Dexamethasone – This drug can be used to prevent AMS either for those who cannot take acetazolamide, or for a forced rapid ascent to very high altitude, such as flying to over 14,000 feet (4,250 meters) on an overnight rescue.

The dosage for adults is 4 mg orally every six hours. Starting the medication two to four hours prior to ascent is probably adequate, although the exact timing for beginning and discontinuing the medication has not yet been established. Discontinuing dexamethasone before acclimatization has taken place may "unmask" the symptoms of AMS.

With short-term use, the side effects from dexamethasone are minimal. Dyspepsia, bizarre dreams, dysphoria, and euphoria occasionally occur.

3. Nifedipine – The prophylactic administration of nifedipine is effective in lowering pulmonary artery pressure and preventing high-altitude pulmonary edema in susceptible individuals. The prophylactic dose of nifedipine is 20 mg every eight hours to be taken during the ascent phase of the expedition and for three additional days at altitude.

Possible side-effects include dizziness, flushing or a feeling of warmth, headache, weakness, nausea, heartburn, muscle cramps, tremors, swelling of the arms or legs, nervousness, mood changes, low blood pressure, and heart palpitations. Long-term efficacy and the effects of withdrawal are not known. Consider the use of this drug for mountain sports only when the most important preventive measure, gradual ascent, has failed, and in patients with a previous history of HAPE.

■ III. GUIDELINES FOR ASSESSMENT AND TREATMENT

Altitude illness is caused by ascending too quickly for an individual's physiology to cope with the hypoxic stress. The treatment of choice for all forms of high-altitude illness is descent. However, mild forms of altitude illness usually resolve spontaneously in two to four days and descent is not necessary. There are few studies of treatment of AMS, and these guidelines reflect expert opinion more than well-controlled research studies. Treatment is based on four principles: 1) stop ascent in presence of symptoms (do not go up unless symptoms go down), 2) descend if there is no improvement or condition worsens, 3) descend immediately if HAPE, loss of coordination, or changes in level of consciousness are present, and 4) ill persons must not be left alone or sent down alone.

A. Acute Mountain Sickness: Individuals with AMS have headache, anorexia, nausea, insomnia, lack of normal diuresis, and lassitude. The syndrome resembles an alcohol hangover. There are no characteristic physical findings. Basic treatment is to descend or to stop ascent and wait for improvement before proceeding. Continuing ascent in the presence of symptoms is ill-advised.

After stopping the ascent, more advanced treatment consists of administering supplemental oxygen (1 L/min at rest), which is especially helpful during sleep. Aspirin or acetaminophen, with codeine if necessary, is useful for headaches. Prochlorperazine or promethazine can be used for nausea. Prochlorperazine 10 mg parenterally or orally every 6 hours, or 25 mg rectally every 12 hours, for an average-size adult, also increases the hypoxic drive to breathe. Promethazine can be administered as 25 mg parenterally, or as 25 or 50-mg suppositories for adults every 8 hours. Use no more than three doses of either drug. Note that both prochlorperazine and promethazine may cause extrapyramidal reactions requiring treatment with diphenhydramine. Treatment of the illness, rather than just the symptoms, requires acetazolamide. This speeds acclimatization and aborts the illness. A response is usually seen within 12 to 24 hours. *If the illness progresses, descent is mandatory.*

B. High-Altitude Pulmonary Edema: Mild HAPE presents with decreased exercise performance, fatigue, dyspnea on exertion but not at rest, a dry cough, and localized rales. In moderate to severe HAPE there is marked weakness and fatigue, cyanosis, a dry to raspy cough, tachypnea after 20 minutes of rest (respiratory rate greater than 20), tachycardia after 20 minutes of rest(heart rate greater than 130), rales, a gurgling sensation in the chest, and late in the course, a productive cough. Neurological symptoms and signs may also be present.

Oxygen, if available, improves arterial oxygenation and lowers pulmonary arterial pressure (PAP). Immediate descent is essential in moderate to severe cases with 2000 to 4000 feet (600 to 1,200 meters) usually being sufficient. Keep the patient warm, because cold raises the PAP. Because exercise raises PAP and lowers arterial oxygenation, exert the patient as little as possible.

Advanced treatment may consist of acetazolamide (250 mg every 6 hours) in mild cases and nifedipine (20 mg stat sublingual, or chew and swallow, followed with 20 mg every 6 hours) in moderate to severe cases. An EPAP mask can be a temporizing measure. In particular, a portable hyperbaric chamber (Gamow Bag®) is highly useful in reversing the effects of high altitude, and can make a non–ambulatory patient ambulatory. Constant monitoring of a patient in a Gamow Bag® is mandatory. Duration of treatment should be until symptoms clear and the weather or climbing conditions permit the aided descent of the patient.

C. High-Altitude Cerebral Edema: Assessment of HACE is based on progressive neurological deterioration, with changes in consciousness and ataxia, accompanied by impaired judgment, hallucinations, severe headache and eventually coma. Basic treatment is immediate descent, until obvious improvement occurs. Initially provide supplemental oxygen starting at 6 liters/minute for the first fifteen minutes, followed by a flow rate of 2 liters/minute. More advanced treatment includes dexamethasone 10 mg intravenously, followed by 4 mg intramascularly every 6 hours until symptoms subside. Response is usually noted within 12 to 24 hours, but descent is still mandatory. Use the Gamow Bag®, if available, as described above.

D. Peripheral Edema: High-altitude may cause swelling of the hands, ankles, or face (usually the periorbital region). Elevate the extremities, if possible. The edema will resolve with descent, or will resolve spontaneously with acclimatization and spontaneous diuresis. Descent is not mandatory unless signs and symptoms of more serious altitude illnesses are present.

CHAPTER TEN

Hypothermia

■ I. GENERAL INFORMATION

Hypothermia, a reduction in core temperature to below 95° Fahrenheit (35°C), can appear rapidly or slowly. **Acute** hypothermia presents with a sudden drop in body core temperature within two hours. This is usually caused by immersion in cold water or a sudden change in the weather. **Chronic** hypothermia is the result of a gradual drop in body core temperature over six hours or longer. Most chronic hypothermia deaths occur when the ambient temperature ranges from 30 to 50°F (−1 to 10°C). Hypothermia is almost always preventable by minimizing heat loss via conduction, convection, radiation,and evaporation. Prevention includes 1) proper choice and use of clothing and shelter, 2) avoidance of overexertion, 3) staying dry (a combination of proper clothing and avoidance of overexertion), 4) maintaining hydration, and 5) adequate nutrition.

A. Mild Hypothermia: Hypothermia is considered mild if the rectal temperature is below 95°F (35°C) and above 90°F (32°C). Taking rectal temperatures in the wilderness, however, is impractical at best, and at worst dangerously exposes the already cold patient. Mild hypothermia almost always first manifests itself as a loss of judgment and fine motor coordination. Shivering is often suppressed by physical activity, but by the time core temperatures reach 95°F (35°C), most patients are shivering uncontrollably. Slurred speech and a stumbling gait are often present. In fact, the development of ataxia is highly suggestive of hypothermia in a cold-exposed patient (or of High Altitude Cerebral Edema at high altitude). It is important to note that most patients with mild hypothermia are still able to rewarm themselves (patients who can shiver can rewarm themselves), although they require protection from further heat loss in order to rewarm.

B. Profound Hypothermia: Hypothermia is considered profound if the rectal temperature drops below 90°F (35°C). Since taking rectal temperatures may not be possible or appropriate, diagnosis is based on profoundly altered mental status and profound loss of coordination. Lassitude, apathy, or an uncooperative attitude are common. Shivering stops, and the patient loses the ability to rewarm. Pupils may be dilated and fixed. The trunk of the body will be cold to touch. The patient may be rigid and unresponsive, with non-palpable pulse and respirations, but not dead. The patient should not be presumed dead unless these conditions persist after warming.

■ II. GUIDELINES FOR FIELD REWARMING

Recognize the severity of hypothermia.

For patients with mild hypothermia, remove the patient from, or limit further exposure to, the environment. As much as possible, protect the patient from wet, wind, and cold. Remove wet clothing as soon as possible and protect from further heat loss, especially covering the head and neck. Insulate the patient from the ground. Rehydrate the patient with warm sweet drinks and feed high-energy foods if the patient is able to swallow. External heat sources, such as chemical heat packs or hot water bottles should not be applied directly to the patient's skin, but can be wrapped in clothing and applied to the neck, armpits, over the kidneys, and to the groin. A patient may be placed in a sleeping bag, ideally two zipped together with one or two normothermic persons, all dressed in dry clothing. Once adequately insulated, the patient may be placed near an external heat source, such as a fire, to add further heat.

Patients with profound hypothermia, must be handled gently while removing wet clothing and performing other life-sustaining measures. Rough movement may cause ventricular fibrillation. Aggressive rewarming, such as warm water immersion, may also cause ventricular fibrillation. Do not rub the extremities. If possible, place the patient in a pre-warmed sleeping bag, well-insulated from the ground, and wrap the patient in a radiation barrier, such as a sheet of plastic or tent fly, to maximize heat conservation. External heat sources, such as heat packs, may be placed inside the barrier as indicated above. Supplemental oxygen, preferably humidified, can be extremely valuable in a severely ill patient. Cuddling with two rescuers, as indicated in mild hypothermia treatment, may be life-saving.

■ III. GUIDELINES FOR EVACUATION

Once a patient with mild hypothermia is adequately rewarmed, with a return to normal mental status, there is no need for evacuation, although take care to prevent a recurrence. If rewarming is not feasible, the monitor the patient while walking out before the problem becomes more profound. Patients who do not respond to rewarming, or who obviously have profound hypothermia, must be "wrapped" for maximum heat retention, and evacuation initiated as soon as possible. It is virtually impossible to rewarm a profoundly hypothermic patient in the field. The prevention of further heat loss requires active intervention. It is dangerous to simply leave the profoundly hypothermic individual in a cold state. Evacuation of such a patient is urgent and must be as gentle as possible to prevent ventricular fibrillation.

CHAPTER ELEVEN

Frostbite/ Immersion Foot

■ I. GENERAL INFORMATION

Frostbite is localized injury or death of tissue from exposure to subfreezing cold. The chance of damage is increased by: 1) temperatures below 28°F (–2°C), and especially temperatures of 20°F (–7°C) or less, 2) high winds, 3) high altitude, 4) use of tobacco, alcohol, or other drugs, 5) contact with heat-conductive materials, such as metal, water, or gasoline, 6) overexertion, which produces fatigue and sweat, 7) previous frostbite injury, and 8) thaw and refreeze of a frostbitten area.

Measures to help prevent frostbite include: 1) avoiding constriction of feet from tight boots or too many pairs of socks in larger boots, 2) preserving heat by keeping head, neck, and face covered, 3) wearing mittens instead of gloves, 4) staying well-hydrated, 5) maintaining metabolic heat production with adequate caloric intake, 6) keeping dry, and 7) avoiding direct skin–metal or skin–fluid contact.

Immersion foot (trenchfoot) is a cold weather, non-freezing injury resulting from vasoconstriction of the arterioles with subsequent loss of heat and oxygen supply to surface tissues.

Prevention includes 1) avoidance of tight-fitting footwear, 2) changing into dry socks regularly (at least once a day), and 3) periodic (every 4 hours in extreme wet and cold conditions)air-drying, elevation, and massaging of feet to promote circulation.

■ II. GUIDELINES FOR ASSESSMENT AND TREATMENT

Superficial frostbite: The skin is pale and cold, but underlying tissues remain soft and pliable. Treat superficial frostbite with passive skin-to-skin contact or rapid rewarming in water no hotter than 108°F (42°C). If a thermometer is not available, the treating person should test the water with his elbow before immersing the frostbitten extremity. The temperature should be similar to a hot tub. After thawing, a few clear fluid-filled blisters may develop in superficial frostbite. Extreme care must be taken with frostbitten tissue to prevent refreezing. Evacuate as soon as possible if blisters have formed. This can be a self-evacuation if the hands are involved, but might require a litter evacuation if the feet are affected.

Deep frostbite involves skin and deep structures, including muscle, tendons, and possibly even bone. The affected part is hard and not pliable. If deep frostbite is diagnosed, evacuate the patient immediately. Patients with frostbitten, unthawed feet may walk to self evacuate. During evacuation, if possible, protect the affected part with dry insulation, such as clean dry socks or dry mittens. Remove jewelry and all constrictive clothing. After evacuation, or if transportation is certain, rapidly rewarm the frostbitten area in water pre-heated to 104 to 108°F (40 to 42° C). After thawing, multiple fluid-filled and hemorrhagic blisters form. The portion of the extremity beyond the hemorrhagic blisters is extremely damaged and may eventually become gangrenous. Suspend the frostbitten area in the container of water without allowing contact with the sides. Check water temperature often. Avoid excessive heat. During thawing, pain is usually severe and analgesics, including narcotics, are indicated. When rewarming is accomplished, dry the affected parts gently, place sterile gauze between digits, and apply aloe vera or antibiotic ointment gently to damaged skin. Elevate the injured part and leave open to the air. Provide definitive medical care as soon as possible. Prior to further transport, provide adequate insulation to the injured part to prevent refreezing. Be especially cautions if evacuating by helicopter to protect the victim from the cold rotor wash.

Early signs of *immersion foot* injury include cold, swollen, waxy feet, mottled with dark burgundy to blue splotches. Skin is sodden and friable. In the later stage, feet become red and hot, and blisters often form. Infection and gangrene frequently result. Field treatment includes 1) maintenance of dry, warm feet, 2) oral hydration, 3) ibuprofen every 6 hours, and 4) immediate evacuation to definitive care (note: walking may be difficult for the patient).

■ III. CONTROVERSIES

A. Should deep frostbite be thawed in the field? There is evidence that the longer tissue stays frozen, the worse the injury. Frozen extremities in an otherwise uninjured patient are difficult to keep frozen, and spontaneous thawing usually occurs during evacuation. Field therapy, which can render an ambulatory patient non–ambulatory, must be balanced against the time required for evacuation.

B. Should a patient self-evacuate on frozen toes/feet prior to thawing if worse freezing is unlikely or field thawing can not be easily accomplished? The longer the extremity is frozen, the greater the tissue damage, although even more significant damage occurs with a thaw followed by freezing. The decision to walk out on frozen feet should not be made if there is any reasonable ability to thaw and provide further protection from freezing. Thawed toes may not be so painful as to preclude self evacuation. Deep frostbite of the entire foot may become so painful and debilitating upon thawing that self evacuation becomes impossible. As the field diagnosis before thawing may be difficult to accurately access, frozen extremities should generally be thawed and protected from further freezing as soon as possible, realizing that the victim might not be able to self-evacuate.

CHAPTER TWELVE

Heat-Related Illnesses

■ I. GENERAL INFORMATION

Heat-related illnesses comprise several conditions caused by exposure to hot environments, or intense exercise in moderate environments, that range from mild discomfort to life-threatening illness. Hyperthermia occurs when heat stress on the body, from internal metabolic heat production and external sources, overcomes the heat dissipating capability of the body. Extreme untreated hyperthermia can rapidly become life threatening.

Heat illnesses are preventable. Prevention includes:

1) Acclimatization, the process by which the body adapts to heat exposure, is induced by a minimum of 60 to 90 minutes of exercise in the heat each day for one to two weeks. Initial adaptation occurs within a few days. The most significant change is an increase in sweat volume initiated at a lower skin temperature. This increases evaporative cooling and results in a lower heart rate and core temperature for a given amount of work in the heat. 2) Hydration with adequate fluid quantities. An acclimatized person can lose 1 to 1.5 liters/hour of sweat during exercise. Relieving thirst alone will not maintain full hydration. Start each work period by drinking 500 ml of water, followed by 200 to 300 ml at least every 20 minutes during exertion. Please refer to the section on Oral Fluid and Electrolyte Replacement, page 38.

3) Dress appropriately in light-colored, loose-fitting clothing, allowing maximum evaporative heat loss.

4) Rest frequently, especially before full acclimatization, preferably in shade, and ideally with a wipe of cool water on exposed areas of skin.

5) Maximize evaporative cooling by dipping clothing periodically in water, if available.

6) Physical fitness improves exercise tolerance in the heat, but it does not acclimatize. Even well trained athletes benefit from acclimatization. The insulation of excess body fat reduces heat loss.

■ II. GUIDELINES FOR ASSESSMENT AND TREATMENT

A. **Heat cramps** are muscle spasms that may be severe, usually in large, heavily exercised muscle groups like legs and abdomen. They are probably caused by a combination of electrolyte depletion, hyperventilation with respiratory alkalosis, and plasma volume depletion. They resolve with rest and oral or intravenous fluids that contain sodium. Cold oral fluids are absorbed more quickly than warm ones. Gentle massage of the cramped muscles is usually beneficial. After recovery, the activity may be resumed, but if the cramps return, a 24-hour rest is recommended.

B. Heat syncope is seen immediately after periods of strenuous work in hot environments. Patients regain consciousness quickly.Treat with recumbent rest in a cooler area and splash water on exposed skin, to enhance cooling. Oral rehydration is indicated when fully alert. Assess the patient for injuries if a fall was associated with the syncope.

C. Heat rash, (prickly heat or miliaria) is an acute inflammatory disease of the skin seen in humid regions following prolonged sweating. Sweat gland ducts become blocked with keratinizing cells and accumulated sweat is forced through the duct walls, inciting inflammation in adjacent soft tissue. Erythematous pruritic papules appear on trunk and extremities, excluding hands and feet. Secondary infection may occur. In severe cases heat tolerance is reduced due to decreased sweating. In the field, keep the affected areas clean and limit exercise and heat exposure.

D. Heat exhaustion is caused by the depletion of salt and/or water. Symptoms and signs include: weakness, inability to work, headache, mild confusion, nausea, faintness, anorexia, dyspnea, and rapid pulse. Skin may be warm or cool with sweating. The core temperature may be normal to moderately elevated. The patient should rest in a cool area and rehydrate orally, preferably with cool, lightly-salted water or an electrolyte solution. The patient may benefit from cooling of the skin by wetting and fanning. When fully recovered, activity may continue, depending on the extent of the illness, recovery may take as long as 24 hours.

E. Heat stroke is a true medical emergency in which elevated core body temperature (above 105°F, 40.5°C, rectal) causes renal, hepatic, and nervous system damage. Persons at an increased risk of heat stroke include those who are obese, unfit, unacclimatized, elderly, acutely ill, dehydrated from vomiting or diarrhea; individuals with underlying medical conditions, such as coronary heart disease and hyperthyroidism; and individuals on certain medications, e.g. beta-blockers, stimulants, diuretics, or anticholinergics.

Skin may be dry or sweaty; sweating is often preserved in fit persons suffering exertional heat stroke. Symptoms and signs include confusion, disorientation, bizarre behavior, ataxia, tachycardia, tachypnea, and hot, red skin.

Both heat stroke and heat exhaustion may present as collapse in the face of a heat load – environmental heat, metabolic heat from exercise, or a combination of both. Both may have altered consciousness, elevated temperatures, and rapid pulse. Heat stroke is differentiated from heat exhaustion by the presence of cardiovascular shock, persistent profound mental status changes, and markedly elevated temperature. In heat exhaustion, mental status and blood pressure normalize rapidly as in syncope, if the patient is recumbent in the shade.

Heat stroke has a high mortality rate. Whenever there is altered mental status and elevated temperature, rapid cooling is essential and must be started in the field. Treatment may include: 1) shading from direct sunlight and removal of excess clothing; 2) wetting with tepid or cool water and fanning aggressively; 3) ice packs at the neck, armpits, and groin; and 4) massage of extremities to return cooler peripheral blood to the core. Do not give antipyretics like aspirin or acetaminophen. If possible, check the rectal temperature every 20 minutes and, when the temperature reaches approximately 100 to 102°F (37.7 to 38.8°C), taper off the cooling efforts, as rapid cooling below this point may lead to shivering. Monitor carefully for rebound temperature increase. If the patient returns to a level of consciousness appropriate for oral hydration, give fluids. Immediate evacuation is indicated.

CHAPTER THIRTEEN

Lightning Injuries

■ I. GENERAL INFORMATION

One bolt of lightning may generate 300,000 amps and 2 billion volts - an awesome power capable of great destructive force. A single strike often injures or kills more than one person. Lightning injures or kills in one of four ways: 1) direct strike, 2) splash after striking a nearby object, 3) ground current, or 4) trauma from the blast of exploding air. Lightning causes serious injury or death in about one-third of its victims and permanent sequelae of some sort in about two–thirds of survivors. The factors related to a fatal outcome include immediate cardiopulmonary arrest or leg or head burns. Because any electrical current takes the shortest path between contact points, multiple organ systems may be injured. The duration of a lightning strike is so brief (less than one millisecond) that it may not penetrate, but "flash over" the patient's skin.

Although lightning strikes are unpredictable, there are ways to reduce the chance of injury. During an electrical storm: 1) avoid open areas where you are one of the tallest objects, 2) do *not* seek shelter under a single tree or bush or rock that stands in an open area, 3) avoid extremes of high or low ground, 4) avoid contact with metal objects unless you can get completely inside of one (such as an enclosed automobile), 5) seek shelter deep in a *dry* cave, staying away from the sides and roof, 6) seek shelter among trees or bushes or rocks of uniform size, 7) if boating, attempt to get to shore, waves and shore–line permitting, 8) squat with your feet close together or sit in a compact position on a non-conductive material, such as a foam pad or rope coil, and 9) spread out a group but stay close enough to maintain visual contact with each other.

■ II. GUIDELINES FOR ASSESSMENT

Victims of lightning strike are not electrically charged and pose no threat to rescuers. Patients typically fall into one of three categories: 1) minimally injured, requiring little immediate care other than psychological support, although they must receive a thorough examination when time allows, 2) seriously injured, often initially unconscious, requiring immediate attention to airway and obvious injuries, including appropriate stabilization for possible head and spine injuries, and 3) maximally injured, in cardiopulmonary arrest, requiring long-term efforts at CPR, which may result in full recovery. Fixed, dilated pupils may be a transient phenomenon. With multiple casualties, unlike normal triage situations, give priority care to those who appear dead after a lightning strike. These victims may be salvaged by CPR. Evacuate all patients surviving a lightning strike for definitive medical evaluation and treatment.

For patients who are not in cardiac arrest, but who are unconscious, consider placing a controlled airway (naso- or endotracheal tube, or cricothyrotomy). Therapy for increased intracranial pressure (see Head and Spinal Injuries) may be necessary.

In patients with cardiac arrest continue aggressive CPR. Investigate for multiple-organ injuries, including cardiac, renal, and CNS injury. Prolonged ventilatory support may be necessary due to brainstem insult, and may result in complete recovery.

Promptly investigate the hypotensive patient for major hemorrhage, spinal shock, or fluid loss from burns. Internal burns of muscles may result in extensive fluid loss, out of proportion to the external burns. Test vision and hearing. Tetanus immunization must be current. Admit patients with major injuries, arrhythmias, mental status, neurological changes, or chest pain to the hospital. Re-examine all patients within 24 hours and advise of the potential for immediate and delayed sequelae, including neuorological, renal, cardiac, and muscular dysfunction.

CHAPTER FOURTEEN

Field Water Disinfection

■ I. GENERAL INFORMATION

Wilderness surface water carries a risk of enteric illness due to ingestion of waterborne pathogens that include bacteria, viruses, protozoan cysts, and some parasitic eggs or larvae. Risk varies with geographic location. In North America, *Giardia lamblia* is the most common microbial contaminant, but *Campylobacter jejuni*, enterotoxigenic *E. coli*, enteric viruses, and *Cryptosporidium* have caused outbreaks of illness. In developing countries, surface and tap water must be considered contaminated. Potential microorganisms include protozoa *(Entamoeba histolytica, Giardia lamblia, Cryptosporidium)*, bacteria *(E. coli, Shigella, Vibrio cholerae, Salmonella, C. jejuni, V. parahaemolyticus)*, viruses (hepatitis A and other enteric viruses), or helminths. Potable water can be prepared by disinfecting water using one of several means.

■ II. METHODS OF WATER DISINFECTION

A. Heat. As in pasteurization, temperatures above 160°F (70°C) kill all enteric pathogens within 30 minutes, and 185°F (85°C) is effective within a few minutes. Thus, disinfection occurs during the time required to heat water from 140°F (60°C) to boiling temperature, so any water brought to a boil, even at high altitudes, is safe. For a margin of safety, boil for one minute or leave covered and hot for several minutes after boiling.

B. Filtration may be used for *Giardia* and other protozoal cysts, enteric bacteria, and parasitic eggs. However, for field use, filtration alone does not adequately remove viruses, although many are removed by adhering to larger particles. The maximum effective filter pore size for Giardia and amoeba cysts is 5 microns. For enteric bacteria, it is 0.2 to 0.5 microns, depending on filter design. *Cryptosporidium* oocysts require less than 3 microns pore size, while other parasitic eggs and larvae are removed with a 20 to 30 micron filter. Most commercial mechanical filters claim removal of *Giardia* and bacteria. Claims for viral removal should be discounted, because they are not well substantiated. Some filters incorporate activated charcoal or an iodine resin. (See Techniques below.)

C. **Clarification** techniques remove suspended particulate matter and many microorganisms. They are not adequate to disinfect water reliably, but may be used to improve clarity and remove organic matter prior to filtration or halogenation.

1. *Sedimentation* is the separation of large particles by gravity. Simply allow water to stand in any container for at least one hour and then decant.

2. *Coagulation, flocculation* (C-F) removes smaller, suspended particles (colloids) that will not settle with simple gravity. This method works best on "cloudy" water, such as brown or green water that is loaded with organic material, as opposed to inorganic matter such as fine clay particles. Alum (aluminum sulfate) is added to water (1/8 to 1/4 tsp/gal) and mixed thoroughly. Then stir or gently agitate occasionally for 5 minutes and allow to settle. Colloidal particles clump together and then settle by gravity or float. The clear water can be decanted, filtered or poured through a cloth or coffee filter. The majority of microorganisms will settle with the floc, but a second disinfection step is recommended. Alum can be obtained at chemical supply stores or some grocery stores (pickling powder). If alum is not available, lime or the fine white ash from a campfire can be used.

3. *Charcoal filters* (purifiers) alone are not adequate for disinfection, although they improve the taste and appearance of water by absorbing chemicals.

D. **Halogens** (chlorine and iodine) are effective disinfectants for viruses, bacteria, and protozoan cysts. Both are available in tablet or liquid form. Iodine also comes in crystalline or polymolecular resin form. In equivalent concentrations, iodine has some advantages over chlorine for field use: less reactivity with organic matter, and less sensitivity to pH.

The effectiveness of a halogen depends on its concentration, the temperature of the water, and the amount of time it is left in the water (contact time). Weaker concentrations or colder water necessitate longer contact time. In the wilderness, the residual concentration cannot be measured, so some uncertainty results. Very high doses of halogen may be used to overcome the uncertainty, but this results in unacceptable taste. Smaller doses are effective in clean water if a prolonged contact time is used. Detection of a faint halogen color, smell or taste indicates the presence of residual halogen in the water.

Because iodine and chlorine react with organic impurities to form a relatively inactive compound, the dose must be increased in grossly contaminated or cloudy water. Inorganic particulate matter does not react with halogens, but can be removed by straining, filtering, sedimentation, or coagulation to improve taste. It is best to clarify water before treatment with halogens. Palatable surface water has a nearly neutral pH, which is optimal for effective treatment with a halogen.

Taste may be improved by several means:

1) Decrease the amount of halogen while increasing contact time.

2) Add flavored drink mix *after* adequate contact time.

3) Pour water through a charcoal filter *after* adequate contact time.

4) Use techniques that do not leave residual halogen, such as heat or filters.

5) Remove the halogen taste by using a zinc brush (see below), sodium thiosulfate, ascorbic acid (vitamin C), or hydrogen peroxide in combination with calcium hypochlorite.

DISINFECTION TECHNIQUES AND HALOGEN DOSES

(All doses added to one quart water: dose/contact time)

Iodination techniques	amount for 4 ppm	amount for 8 ppm

Iodine tabs
tetraglycine hydroperiodide
   EDWGT (emergency drinking water
   germicidal tablet)
   Potable Aqua
   Globaline
	1/2 tab	1 tabs

2% iodine solution (tincture)	0.2 ml 5 gtts	0.4 ml 10 gtts
10% povidone–iodine solution	0.35 ml 8 gtts	0.70 ml 16 gtts
Saturated iodine crystals in water (commercial name: Polar Pure)	13 ml	26 ml
Saturated iodine crystals in alcohol	0.1 ml amount for 5 ppm	0.2 ml amount for 10 ppm
Halazone tabs mono–dichloraminobenzoic acid	2 tabs	4 tabs
household bleach 5% Sodium hypochlorite	0.1 ml 2 gtts	0.2 ml 4 gtts

Concentration of halogenon	Contact time in minutes at various water temperatures		
	5 C	15 C	30 C
2 ppm	240	180	60
4 ppm	180	60	45
8 ppm	60	30	15

Note: Recent data indicate that very cold water requires prolonged contact time with iodine or chlorine to kill Giardia cysts. These contact times in cold water have been extended from the usual recommendations to account for this and for the uncertainty of residual concentration.

■ III. TECHNIQUES FOR WATER DISINFECTION

A. Iodine resins. The resin releases iodine on contact that binds to microorganisms. The exact mechanism of iodine transfer to organisms is not known. Minimal iodine dissolves in water: effluent contains 0.5 to 2.0 ppm iodine. This dissolved iodine is not responsible for disinfection, so many filters include a charcoal resin to remove all iodine dissolved in the water after passing through the iodine resin. Some devices incorporate a 1 micron filter to remove cysts that are resistant to iodine (*Cryptosporidium*), or require longer contact times (*Giardia*). Potential problems include channeling of water through the resin, which may allow some organisms through without contacting the iodine resin.

(Commercial products: PentaPure® from Water Technologies Corporation, and PUR® from Recovery Engineering.)

B. Chlorination-dechlorination. This technique uses very high concentrations of chlorine for disinfection, then "dechlorination" with peroxide, which forms soluble calcium chloride, a tasteless and odorless compound. Excess peroxide bubbles off as oxygen. The kit consists of chlorine crystals (calcium hypochloride) and 30% hydrogen peroxide in separate small Nalgene® bottles. This is a very good technique for highly polluted or cloudy waters, for disinfecting large volumes, and for storing water on boats. Note: 30% peroxide is extremely corrosive and burns skin.

(Commercial product: Sierra Water Purifier®.)

C. Flocculation-chlorination. Tablets contain both alum as a flocculent and chlorine for a disinfectant. This has the advantage of cleaning and disinfecting cloudy or foul smelling water in a one-step process.

The tablet is designed to leave 8 ppm free residual chlorine after flocculation, but 3 to 5 ppm is more common. Extend the recommended 15 minute contact time for added safety in cold water.

(Commercial product: AquaCure®.)

D. Dehalogenation. A small wand with brush-like zinc and copper alloy bristles is used to stir the water to dechlorinate. It is intended to be used after halogenation. Zinc catalyses an electrochemical reaction reducing hypochlorite to chloride or iodine to iodide, neither of which have taste, small, or color. Zinc is not used up so the life span of the product is indefinite. The device is practical only for small amounts of water at a time. Larger volumes or higher concentrations require a considerable amount of time.

(Commercial product: Cl–Out®.)

Very small amounts of sodium thiosulfate or ascorbic acid will accomplish the same chemical reduction, removing halogen taste. These techniques should only be used after adequate contact time.

■ IV. CONTROVERSIES

A. What is the best technique? The best technique depends on personal preference and intended use. Use of heat may be limited by fuel supplies. If planned for a large group, halogenation or high-capacity filters work best. Two-stage techniques are more effective as water quality deteriorates.

Iodine and chlorine have similar antimicrobial activity, although there may be some advantages to iodine. Most prefer the taste of iodine over chlorine in equipotent doses, and iodine is less reactive with nitrogenous wastes in the water. However, iodine is physiologically active, and may be unsafe for individuals with iodine allergies, for those with uncontrolled thyroid disease, and for prolonged use in pregnant women. Although not proven dangerous in healthy individuals, iodine use should be limited to months, not years.

Filtration is not a reliable method of removing viruses. Although viral contamination is currently unlikely in North American alpine surface water, high levels of viral contamination should be assumed in lowland rivers with towns upstream and in developing countries. In these areas, halogenation or heat should be used instead of, or in addition to, filtration.

B. Is *Cryptosporidium* a sufficient risk to mandate filtration of surface water? *Cryptosporidium* is a protozoan, transmitted by the fecal-oral route, that can cause enteric illness. It produces a hardy oocyst. Waterborne outbreaks have been demonstrated and the oocysts have been found to be widespread in surface water. Although pathogenicity is not debated, the epidemiology of infection, specifically the incidence of symptomatic infection and presence of immunity, is unclear. The problem is that the oocyst is extremely resistant to halogens. If this organism is demonstrated to be a common cause of traveler's diarrhea and enteric illness in wilderness travelers, filtration will be an essential step in water disinfection.

C. Are waterborne pathogens a significant source of illness for wilderness and foreign travelers? The major source of traveler's diarrhea is food borne. However, waterborne outbreaks of most enteric pathogens have been confirmed, and the waterborne route has been shown to be a major source of giardiasis outbreaks in the United States, especially from surface water. While the risk of illness from wilderness water in North America may be small and considered negligible by some, countries without sanitation have a much higher risk due to high levels of enteric pathogens in surface water.

CHAPTER FIFTEEN

Oral Fluid and Electrolyte Replacement

■ I. GENERAL INFORMATION

Oral rehydration/electrolyte solutions (ORS) are useful in three circumstances when fluids and electrolytes may be lost in significant amounts: 1) heavy, prolonged exercise with high-volume sweat losses, 2) treatment of mild to moderate heat illness, and 3) illness with diarrhea and/or vomiting. Significant hemorrhage also requires fluid replacement.

A. Fluid replacement during exercise. Large fluid losses may occur during exercise in heat and at high altitudes. Sweat losses of 1 L/h are common during moderate exercise in a hot, environment or at high levels of exertion in a temperate environment. The rate is individual, and depends on the degree of heat acclimatization. Dehydration disposes to heat illness. In high altitude mountaineering, the scarcity of surface water, difficulty adjusting clothing to changing levels of exertion or weather conditions, and respiratory fluid losses from hyperventilation in dry, cold air (averages 1.5 L/day for moderate exertion at 15,000 feet [4,500 meters]) commonly creates fluid needs of 7 to 8 L/day. Dehydration in this environment disposes to altitude sickness, hypothermia, frostbite and venous thrombosis.

During exercise, fluid replacement is essential. Minimal water recommendations for hard exertion are 500 ml before and 200 to 300 ml every 20 minutes during exercise. People without regular access to water should rehydrate at every opportunity, and gauge hydration by volume and color of urine.

Sweat contains electrolytes: sodium (average 20 to 60 mEq/L), chloride, and small amounts of potassium. In most instances, replacement of electrolytes during sweat loss is not necessary, so ORS have no advantage over plain water. Electrolyte needs can usually be met by regular meals and snacks, which also provide more calories than electrolyte solutions.

In endurance events or work/exercise for more than two hours in a very hot environment with high sweat losses, electrolyte supplements are recommended. During exercise, a solution containing 2 to 6% glucose and 30 mEq/L sodium is optimal to maintain palatability. Higher glucose concentrations may delay gastric emptying and promote osmotic diarrhea, but new long-chain carbohydrates that break down to simple sugars during digestion can provide larger amounts of sugar. Excessive sodium can cause nausea. Do not ingest salt tablets directly because they can cause gastric irritation and vomiting. One or two salt tablets, however, can be dissolved in a liter of water. Commercial sports drinks contain about 6% glucose and 10 to 25 mEq/L of sodium. Simple solutions can be made at home. One tsp/L sugar yields a 0.35 to 0.5% solution, so 3 to 4 tsp sugar in a liter yields a 1 to 2% solution with about 50 kcal. One-half tsp NaCl (table salt) added to 1 liter of water yields about 30 mEq/L. In the wilderness, it is convenient to replace salt with snack foods during exertion. Although the teaspoon measurement method is quite variable (yielding 3.5 to 5.0 cc), concentrations over the resulting range are not dangerous.

B. Treatment of mild heat illness. Oral electrolyte solutions are an excellent means of treating mild to moderate forms of heat illness, such as heat syncope, heat cramps, and heat exhaustion. The patient must rest in the shade and sip fluids. Usually 1 to 2 liters of fluids similar to exercise replacement fluids are adequate. Oral fluids cannot be used for heat stroke with altered consciousness, unless via a naso–gastric tube.

C. Replacement of enteric fluid losses. Diarrheal illness (e.g. traveler's diarrhea) is the main indication for oral electrolyte solutions. Most cases of infectious enteritis are self-limited – although antibiotics can shorten the duration of most bacterial enteric infections. The major morbidity from these infections results from dehydration, so rehydration and maintenance of fluids and electrolytes are essential. Diarrheal fluid contains more electrolytes than sweat: sodium (50 to 100 mEq/L), chloride, and significant amounts of potassium and bicarbonate. Oral replacement is feasible because the gut can absorb water and electrolytes when administered with glucose, even during severe secretory diarrhea.

The optimal composition of rehydration fluid for gastrointestinal losses is a sodium concentration between 50 and 90 mEq/L. The lower concentration may be more palatable, but the higher concentration is most effective with moderate dehydration. Maximal glucose concentration is 2 to 2.5%. Higher concentrations may have an osmotic effect, making diarrhea worse. Cereal-based ORS contains complex carbohydrate molecules from rice or grains that do not create an excessive osmotic load, but are digested as simple glucose. At least 20 mEq/L of potassium is necessary and 30 mEq/L of bicarbonate is optimal.

The World Health Organization (WHO) has developed electrolyte salts specifically for diarrheal illness that contain 90 mEq of sodium, 20 mEq of potassium, 80 mEq of chloride, 30 mEq of bicarbonate or trisodium citrate, and 111 mmol (2%) of glucose, which must be mixed with 1 liter of disinfected water. Packets of these oral rehydration salts are distributed throughout the world by WHO and UNICEF, commonly under the name Oralyte. In the United States, the WHO salts are hard to find [manufactured and distributed by Jianas Brothers, Kansas City, MO]. The International Association for Medical Assistance to Travelers (IAMAT) can provide ORS salt packets for a nominal donation [417 Center St., Lewistown, NY 14092, (716) 754-4883]. More expensive premixed solutions are available, but are not practical for wilderness or foreign travel. Sports drinks and other "clear liquids" contain insufficient sodium and potassium and excessive glucose for treatment of diarrheal induced dehydration, but are better than plain water.

If pre-measured salts are not available, a substitute recommended by the Centers for Disease Control and Prevention (CDC) consists of alternating glasses of the following two fluids:

> Glass #1: 8 oz fruit juice (such as apple, orange, or lemon)
> 1/2 tsp honey or corn syrup
> 1 pinch salt
> Glass #2: 8 oz water (boiled or treated)
> 1/4 tsp baking soda

However, these ingredients may not be available to remote travelers.

Plain salt and sugar solutions, similar to those used for heat/exercise replacement, can be used for mild dehydration, but are not adequate for serious dehydration or replacement of continuing high losses. For mild dehydration, partial maintenance, or supplementation, or where nothing else is available, rice water, fruit juice, coconut milk, or diluted cola drinks may suffice.

■ II. GUIDELINES FOR FLUID REPLACEMENT

Achieve replacement of estimated fluid deficit in about four hours by giving 50 ml/kg body weight for mild dehydration and 100 ml/kg for moderate dehydration. This means that for mild dehydration, an adult should drink 250 ml of oral rehydration solution every 30 minutes for the first 4 to 6 hours. Children should drink 200 to 250 ml/hour. In addition, they may drink water as desired. Give infants under 3 months a 100 ml dose each hour with every third dose replaced by plain water. Ingestion of frequent, small amounts, rather than rapid ingestion, minimizes vomiting. Fluid deficit is replaced within 12 hours in 90% of patients. Determine maintenance fluids by estimating or measuring stool losses plus normal maintenance requirements. Since this is not often possible in the field, give 10 to 15 ml/kg body weight/diarrheal stool.

At least 90% of patients during diarrhea epidemics can be successfully rehydrated using only ORS. Failure of ORS occurs when stool losses exceed oral intake. Vomiting, unless frequent and protracted, does not preclude rehydration with oral solutions. Fluids may be administered by nasogastric tube when the patient is unable or unwilling to drink adequate fluids. Intravenous fluids can be reserved for the initial hydration of patients with shock, obtundation, seizures, or intractable vomiting. When IV fluids are necessary, ORS usually can be initiated within 4 hours and exclusively used within 24 hours.

■ III. CONTROVERSIES

A. Does ORS cause hypernatremia in patients without cholera? Many physicians in developed countries avoid ORS because of an unsubstantiated concern for hypernatremia in small children. This concern has led to lower sodium concentrations (50 to 75 mEq/L) in commercial ORS sold in the United States and recommendations to use the higher concentration only for initial rehydration then lower concentrations for maintenance. This complexity can be avoided if plain water or formula is alternated with ORS in the maintenance phase of treatment.

B. Are electrolyte replacement drinks necessary for wilderness activities? Cases of severe hyponatremia in endurance athletes and recreational hikers in hot climates have been reported, and were probably caused by water intoxication. As sweat losses increase with environmental heat stress and prolonged exercise, electrolyte replacement becomes more important. Most wilderness sports such as hiking, climbing, or skiing offer frequent opportunities to rest and ingest food and fluids. If snack foods are eaten regularly, plain water will be safe for fluid replacement. Unfortunately, many hikers favor snack foods that are high in carbohydrates and fats (such as candy) but low in sodium. Some individuals, noting the edema present in their hands and feet associated with heat or altitude exposure, attempt to restrict their sodium intake. The development of heat exhaustion causes nausea, preventing food intake. If frequent snack and meal breaks are not planned, electrolyte replacement fluids are recommended for sustained wilderness activities in hot climates.

CHAPTER SIXTEEN

Wild Land Animal Attacks

■ I. GENERAL INFORMATION

Although few truly large and wild animals remain in the contiguous United States, injuries from attacks by alligators, bison, bears and cougars (mountain lions) occur annually. In Alaska and overseas, wild animal attacks are a more significant cause of morbidity and mortality. Many of these involve predation by the big cats or by bears, but other species such as elephant, rhinoceros, wild pigs or hippopotamus also attack humans.

Injuries from wild animal attack result from a variety of mechanisms, including biting, clawing, chewing, goring, tossing or trampling. As a result the victim often sustains major trauma far beyond a simple bite, involving multiple organ systems and locations. Wounds are always contaminated with oral or soil pathogens.

A. Wild Cats: Wild cats spring from behind to attack the neck of their prey, sharply hyperextending the neck to fracture the cervical spine and transecting the spinal cord and great vessels with their teeth.

B. Horned animals: Goring injuries from animals such as bull, American buffalo, bison, elephant or rhinoceros produce deep puncture wounds. These may rip along fascial planes or penetrate deeply; evisceration is common. Trampling or tossing by these animals also results in blunt trauma to the victim.

C. Bears: Bears of all types claw, bite, crush and tear their victims. Attacks are often aimed preferentially at the head, with extensive facial injuries and scalping. Chewing on extremities is also frequently described.

■ II. PREVENTION

For all wild animal attacks, prevention can be summarized as "don't get too close: stay out of the way." Approaching too closely while photographing is particularly risky. Alertness and awareness of the animal habitat in which you are traveling will prevent many encounters. There is safety in numbers. Group travel is safer than solo travel.

General recommendations in case of an attack or encounter include attempting to remove the perceived threat to the animal (i.e. yourself). In an unanticipated wild animal encounter, slowly and quietly back away. Running or fleeing will elicit a predatory response. "Playing dead" by dropping to the ground, rolling into a knee-to-chest ball and covering your head and face with your arms is advised in a sudden grizzly encounter. These maneuvers all "remove the threat."

If an attack is unprovoked, with human seen as prey, aggressively fighting back is recommended. Behavior such as advancing rather than fleeing, making loud noises, or waving arms to appear larger and more threatening may forestall an attack. Vigorous resistance with physical fighting, including striking the attacking animal with fists or any object or weapon, has been effective in repelling attacks by cougars, lions, tigers, brown and black bears and even crocodiles. Cayenne pepper spray may be a useful deterrent if approached by a bear. Many people carry firearms in "bear country." Both pepper spray and firearms may provide a false sense of security. Both must be used correctly by persons trained in their use to be effective.

Avoidance is best. Care in traveling, in camping, food storage, cooking and sleeping arrangements, and preparation with a plan of action in case of an attack is common sense.

■ III. ASSESSMENT AND TREATMENT
Assume all victims of large wild animal attacks have sustained multiple trauma. Beyond the obvious bite, claw or goring wounds, the victim needs assessment for fractures, neurovascular damage, and internal head, chest or abdominal injury. Try to determine the mechanism of injury. Soft tissue damage far beyond the obvious may result from trampling, butting or tossing with ground impact. Bites regularly penetrate more deeply than apparent. Recognize the factor of psychological trauma, even in the field.

Scene security is an initial consideration for rescuers: is the animal gone, or liable to attack again? Do not spend time tracking the attacking animal unless adequate assistance to the victim is simultaneously available and rescuers are experienced and competent in such activity.

ABCs are first as always. Airway management may be complicated with head, facial, neck or chest injuries. Bleeding is controlled by direct pressure. Wash and irrigate wounds with the cleanest water available. Filter or boil if this can be quickly accomplished. Remove debris or foreign bodies (see section on wilderness wound management.) Wound cleaning is the single most important step in preventing infection: its importance cannot be overemphasized.

Use the cleanest available material for bandaging. Splint large open wounds or lacerations as well as suspected fractures. Cover abdominal eviscerations or eye injuries with a moist clean dressing: evacuate immediately.

Blunt trauma mandates evaluation for cervical spine injury, closed head injury, intraperitoneal bleeding and internal chest trauma. Multiple rib fractures with pneumothoraces, pelvic and skull fractures, subdural hematoma, and splenic rupture have been reported with wild animal attacks. Provide supportive care preceding evacuation.

Do not close animal bite or claw wounds, particularly punctures, in the field. Devitalized, necrotic tissue from bite and crush injuries is common, requiring debridement. These injuries are all contaminated. Give parenteral antibiotics, such as a cephalosporin, if available. All wild cats, from cougars in the Western USA and Canada to leopards, lions and tigers in Africa and Asia, inflict bite wounds contaminated with *Pasteurella multocida*. Parenteral antibiotic treatment is indicated with penicillin, or if penicillin allergic, a cephalosporin.

The CDC recommends rabies prophylaxis for "all large wild carnivore" bites. When appropriate administer rabies immune globulin with rabies vaccine as soon as possible. Update tetanus prior to travel as these injuries are high risk wounds for tetanus. Consider rabies prophylaxis for high risk travelers planning long stays in rabies endemic, remote areas.

■ IV. GUIDELINES FOR EVACUATION

Victims of large wild animal attack, even with stable vital signs, usually require emergent evacuation from the field for surgical wound treatment, as well as multiple trauma evaluation with diagnostic studies such as X–ray or CT scans. Lesser wounds or bites may require evacuation for antibiotic treatment, rabies prophylaxis, cosmetic closure or wound exploration and cleaning.

If rescue and evacuation will require days versus hours, close observation of vitals signs, daily wound care with additional field irrigation, cleaning, debridement and dressing change as needed and antibiotic administration is advised.

CHAPTER SEVENTEEN

Reptile Envenomations

■ I. GENERAL INFORMATION

There are approximately 300,000 human snakebites worldwide each year from 2700 known species. In the United States it is estimated that there are 45,000 bites of humans with 8000 envenomations and 5 to 12 deaths per year. Venomous snakes found in the United States include representatives from the family Crotalidae (pit vipers, including rattlesnakes, cottonmouths, and copperheads) and the family Elapidae (which includes coral snakes). There are about 3000 known species of lizards, but only members of the family Helodermatidae (including Gila monsters) are considered venomous. They are found exclusively in the southwestern United States and Mexico. Lizards rarely cause human fatalities. Fatalities from U.S. crotalid envenomation are not common, but complications may be severe.

A. Pit Vipers: Crotalids have a triangular head, cat-like vertical pupils, hinged fangs, and a heat-sensitive "pit" on each side of the head between the tip of the nose and the eye. Rattlesnakes have a variable number of rattles depending upon age and number of molts. They sometimes strike without rattling. About 60% of this country's venomous bites are attributed to rattlesnakes. Cottonmouths (water moccasins) and copperheads are the other two commonly encountered North American pit vipers. Copperhead and cottonmouth venoms are quite similar and weaker than most rattlesnake venoms. Bites by cottonmouths tend to be more serious than copperhead bites because it is a bigger snake.

B. Coral Snakes: The several species of coral snakes are brightly colored, with black noses and alternating red-yellow-red-black bands around their bodies (remember "red on yellow can kill a fellow"). They have relatively small mouths with fixed fangs. From southern Mexico through tropical South America the rules for distinguishing coral snakes are highly unreliable. Unless you are a knowledgeable herpetologist, it is best not to pick up colorful snakes in tropical America.

C. Gila Monsters: These lizards are not large, seldom reaching 20 inches in length. They have blunt heads, beady eyes, and powerful digging claws on short legs. They are shy and appear sluggish, but are capable of swift, determined lunges when threatened or handled.

■ II. PREVENTION:

Wilderness travelers are rarely bitten by venomous reptiles. Avoid reptile bites by: 1) staying away from infested areas; 2) not hiking during times of peak reptile activity (usually at night); 3) watching clearly where one steps; 4) never reaching into concealed areas (gathering firewood at night for example); 5) checking bedding, clothing, and footwear before use; 6) and never handling a venomous reptile, even if it is presumed dead (reflex allows some pit vipers to strike even after death). The chance of envenomation from a strike can be minimized by wearing high leather boots and long pants. Envenomation is more apt to occur in persons who are intoxicated and in young children. It is helpful to know the distribution, markings, and characteristics of venomous reptiles in intended areas of wilderness travel.

■ III. GUIDELINES FOR ASSESSMENT AND TREATMENT

A. Pit Vipers: As many as 20 to 30% of crotalid bites cause no envenomation. Most, but not all, crotalid envenomations result in immediate pain at the bite site, and a rapid onset (within 10 to 15 minutes) of swelling and ecchymosis. Rarely, signs of envenomation are delayed for several hours. Typical paired fang wounds are not always present. A single puncture or a scratch may be the only mark, and the degree of envenomation does not correlate with the size, quality, and number of fang marks.

Assessment of envenomation by a pit viper is the first step in managing a bite in the field. Mark the advancing border of edema and sequentially measure and mark the circumference at the site and at least one location above the bite to detect spreading edema. Reassess these measurements every 15 minutes. Gently cleanse the area. Apply a sterile or clean dressing. The basic tenet is to provide calm, rapid transport to a medical facility. For an upper extremity bite, splint the limb. Do not use pressure dressings, tourniquets, applications of cold, electric shocks, or incisions of the bite site, as these techniques have no known efficacy. Lymphatic constricting bands (barely indenting the skin) are advocated by some, although their use has not been proven to have any definite advantage in pit viper envenomations. The only scientifically proven method for extracting venom from a bite site is with the Extractor® device (Sawyer Products). In animal studies, it has been demonstrated that up to 30% of total injected venom can be removed if the device is used three minutes after the bite occurs.

Encourage the patient to rest and stay calm. Keep the extremity at heart level or lower. Walking out may be attempted if the hike is not too strenuous and the patient is physically and emotionally able to ambulate. Walking out is imperative if the patient is alone. Severe manifestations of poisoning may not occur for several hours, so travel is possible in most cases.

For those with the skill and equipment, use of oxygen is recommended, as is one large-bore (16 g or larger) IV in an unaffected limb. Start at least two large-bore IVs in a patient presenting with shock. Administer either normal saline or Ringer's lactate solution (LR) to support systolic blood pressure above 90 mm Hg. Intubation or vasopressors are rarely necessary in crotalid envenomations. *Field use of intravenous antivenom is not recommended.*

B. Coral Snakes: Elapid envenomations show few immediate symptoms, but may cause respiratory arrest eight to ten hours later when the neurotoxin takes effect. Elapid bites are not as easily assessed for envenomation because there is no significant local tissue injury, systemic signs and symptoms may be delayed for a few hours, and fang marks may not be present. Assume envenomation in coral snake bites, and rapidly evacuate. Follow the recommendations for management of a pit viper envenomation with one exception: place a wide elastic wrap over the bite site. Encounters with coral snakes are rare, and fatal encounters are extremely rare.

C. Gila Monsters: Gila monsters have no injection mechanism for their venom, but they have very powerful jaws and they chew and tear at their victims, drooling venom and producing a substantial amount of pain. Envenomation produces pain, swelling, vomiting, increased heart rate, vertigo, shortness of breath, and loss of consciousness. Follow the recommendations for pit viper envenomation. Fatal Gila monster encounters are extremely rare.

CHAPTER EIGHTEEN

Arthropod Envenomations

■ I. GENERAL INFORMATION

In the United States, arthropods (invertebrates with jointed legs and segmented bodies) cause more deaths by envenomation than reptiles. The most common significant envenomations are caused by Hymenoptera (bees, wasps, etc.), the Arachnida (spiders and scorpions), and Chilopoda (centipedes).

Neither *Latrodectus* (black widow) nor *Loxosceles* (Brown recluse) are aggressive toward humans. These spiders live in crevices under ground cover, trash piles, barns, porches, and outside toilets. Prevention includes inspection, clearing, and care, especially around these areas. Nearly half of all bites could be prevented if toilets and clothing were inspected prior to use.

■ II. GUIDELINES FOR ASSESSMENT AND TREATMENT

A. Stinging Insects: The most common insect stings are from the Hypmenoptera. Although it takes about 300 to 500 stings to make a lethal dose of the complex venom, hypersensitivity, which occurs in approximately 1% of the general public, may result in a life-threatening anaphylactic reaction from a solitary sting. This is more common in adults than in children.

The Hymenoptera comprise four families: 1) honeybees, which account for the most stings and leave the stinger attached to their victims, 2) bumblebees, 3) hornets, yellow jackets, and wasps and 4) fire ants, whose alkaloid venom results in a sterile, burning, vesicular lesion.

Nearly all Hymenoptera stings result in local pain, swelling, and redness. The honeybee stinger should be flicked or scraped out in such a manner to avoid compression of the poison sac, which may result in the injection of still more venom. The site may be treated locally with gentle cleansing, application of cold, elevation, and immobilization. Calm the patient. Common remedies, such as applying a slurry of baking soda or meat tenderizer, often reduce pain. Commercial "sting sticks" containing a topical anesthetic like lidocaine may be used unless the patient is known to be allergic to the drug. Oral aspirin or ibuprofen usually help control pain. The use of a non-invasive suction cup, the Sawyer Extractor®, helps alleviate pain and is effective in removing a portion of the venom if applied within three minutes.

Patients with serious allergic reactions have pruritus, hives, angioedema, and breathing problems. For these individuals apply a light constrictive band (not a tourniquet) proximal to the site. Oral antihistamines (such as diphenhydramine) may be helpful. If the patient is carrying injectable epinephrine, help him or her administer it. Arrange for evacuation as soon as possible. Maintaining ABC's may be extremely difficult without advanced knowledge and equipment.

If any signs of anaphylactic reaction are identified, rescuers carrying epinephrine should administer the drug subcutaneously (0.3 to 0.5 mg for and adult, 0.01 mg/KG up to the adult maximum for a child) or via pre-loaded syringes as often as necessary, depending on the patient's status.

B. Spider Bites: There are approximately 100,000 species of spiders worldwide, with a density of up to two million spiders per acre in some areas. In the United States, the most significant venomous spiders are the black widow (*Latrodectus mactans*) and the fiddleback, or brown recluse (*Loxosceles reclusa*). The venoms of these spiders are potent toxins with numerous antigenic components capable of causing either a systemic manifestation or a local venom reaction.

(1)"Black widow" is itself a misnomer because only three of the five species of widow spider (Family Therdiidae) are actually black, the others being brown and gray. The female spider is the larger of the sexes, often measuring 1 to 1.5 cm long, with a leg span of 4 to 5 cm. The female has a unique hourglass mark, usually red, on the ventral abdominal surface. Newly–hatched spiders are almost entirely red, darkening with progressive molts. Males are 3 to 5 mm long with white stripes along the lateral aspect of the abdomen.

Only adult females can envenomate. The bite usually feels like a mild pinprick, with subsequent slight redness that usually disappears within a few minutes to an hour. Systemic symptoms of envenomation begin 10 to 60 minutes after the bite of the female and are caused by the release of the neurotransmitters acetylcholine and norepinephrine. A few minutes after the bite a small weal appears, followed within 15 to 60 minutes by a band of excruciating cramping pain that remains localized or spreads to involve the thigh, shoulder, back and abdominal muscles. A board-like abdomen often simulates an acute abdomen. Bites on the arm can produce chest pain that mimics a myocardial infarction. Hypertension, respiratory distress, seizures, and, occasionally in the very young or old, cardiopulmonary arrest are all possible. These symptoms frequently subside in 24 hours, but in a few cases recur for several days to months. The very young, very old, and those with hypertension have the greatest risk of morbidity from *Latrodectus* envenomation.

Reassure the patient and have him or her rest as much as possible. Assess ABCs and monitor vital signs. Attempt to assess whether the individual was indeed bitten by a spider or whether another process is occurring. If significant pain is present, immobilize the involved extremity. Oral analgesics are useful for muscle pain.

If available, narcotics may be necessary for pain control, but care must be taken to avoid hypotension and respiratory depression. If IV access can be gained, a muscle relaxant such as methocarbamol may be used as an alternative (1 gram IV slowly over 5 min, followed by 1 gram/250 mL D5W at 100 mL/hr drip). Intravenous calcium gluconate often gives relief from the pain and other symptoms of an *Latrodectus* bite, although the injection may need to be repeated. Immediate evacuation is recommended for signs of serious envenomation.

(2) Fiddlebacks are often called brown recluses, but these spiders are not always distinctively brown. They all have a distinctive violin or fiddle-shaped mark on the dorsal cephalothorax. They average 12 mm long with a leg span of up to 5 cm. The bite of both sexes is equally venomous, although usually painless. Within a few hours, a macule or vesicle may appear at the site. In a severe bite, erythema and blistering follow within 6 to 12 hours. The classic picture is a hemorrhagic vesicle surrounded by a white or pale ischemic zone, and then by an erythematous region - the so-called bull's-eye lesion. By inspection of the lesion alone, however, it is usually impossible to differentiate a *Loxosceles* bite from many other skin lesions and bites. Pruritus and rash can also occur. Nausea, vomiting, headache, and fever are common systemic symptoms. The lesion either resolves or becomes necrotic and indurated. This may require excision or grafting. Symptoms of envenomation with fiddleback bites are caused by cell and tissue injury and direct lytic action of sphingomyelinase on red cell membranes. Rarely, and mostly in children, massive intravascular hemolysis develops after necrosis of the local bite. Deaths have been reported in the United States.

Treatment consists of local wound care. If the wound becomes necrotic and extends to more than 1 cm in diameter, the use of oral dapsone may be indicated. There are potential complications and the efficacy of this treatment has been seriously questioned. The short term application of ice packs to the bite site is as effective as any other form of therapy. While not of proven efficacy, it has virtually no complications and works well. The patient may be placed on a corticosteroid, such as prednisone 1 mg/kg daily for five days, during the acute phase.

C. Scorpion Stings: Approximately 650 species of scorpions inhabit the world, mainly distributed in tropical and subtropical areas. An estimated 40 of these species live in the United States, distributed across 75% of the country but concentrated in the warmer regions. All scorpions inject venom through a single sharp stinger at the tip of the "tail," which is actually an extension of the abdomen. Contact with scorpions is usually accidental. They feed at night. During the daytime they may take shelter in clothing, boots, and bedding. Outdoors, they may often be found under rocks and logs. Checking their hiding places in known scorpion areas is good advice for any traveler. Although the sting is painful, few species inject sufficient venom to be of concern to humans. The only potentially lethal U.S. scorpion is *Centruroides sculpturatus* (*exilicauda* to some taxonomists). *C. gertschi* is generally considered a variety of *sculpturatus*. This scorpion is found in the Southwest, primarily Arizona. It is most active May through August, hibernating in winter. Since specific identification is difficult, the traveler is advised to inquire locally about what dangerous species are present before traveling into scorpion territory. As with Blackwidow spiders, most deaths and serious reactions from *Centruroides* stings are in small children, the elderly, and hypertensives.

Any sting typically produces a burning pain, minimal swelling, redness, vesicles, numbness, tingling, and, uncommonly, weakness or numbness of the affected extremity. *Centruroides* stings are usually acutely painful, with a hypersensitive zone soon developing around the site. The injured area may be sensitive to touch, pressure, heat, and cold. Salivation, diaphoresis, perioral paresthesia, dysphagia, gastric distention, hyperactivity, diplopia, nystagmus, visual loss, incontinence, penile erection, exaggerated reflexes, abdominal pain, opisthotonos, seizures, hypertension (more common), hypotension (less common), pulmonary edema, coma, and muscle paralysis (including respiratory paralysis) can ensue especially, in children. Most non-lethal symptoms last less than four hours.

Treatment includes evaluation and application of cold to the sting site. Clean the site and apply a sterile, or at least clean, dressing. For severe pain, splint or immobilize the affected extremity. Oral, non-narcotic analgesics may be useful. If serious symptoms develop (see above), immediate evacuation is indicated. If possible, bring the scorpion along on the evacuation, but avoid direct handling.

For those with the skill and equipment, benzodiazepine or phenobarbital may be used for seizures and excitability. Methocarbamol may be administered IV for severe muscle spasms. Oral or parenteral antihypertensive medications (such as clonidine) may be required. If there are profound cholinergic effects, administer atropine. Give IV fluids carefully, if needed, since pulmonary edema may develop. Observe all healthy adults for at least four hours after a sting. Admit to the hospital all children and elderly patients stung by scorpions.

Administer IV antivenin only in cases of severe poisoning. It is available in most areas where dangerous scorpions exist. In the United States, it is only available in Arizona. Test for sensitivity to the serum only if the antivenin is to be used. Administer tetanus immunization.

D. Centipede Bites: Centipedes are found all over the United States. They rarely cause serious injury to humans. The giant desert centipede, which may attain a length of 15 cm (6 inches), can give a painful bite. Most bite reactions are local and no fatalities have been documented, but renal failure has been reported. Generally, centipedes hide in dark places. Check shoes, clothing, and bedding before use while traveling in centipede-infested areas.

Local reactions to centipede bites, in addition to intense pain, may include edema and erythema. Manifestations last 4 to 12 hours. In severe bites, tenderness may persist or recur. To prevent secondary infection, cleanse the wound with soap and water. Apply cold and/or give oral analgesics for pain. In more serious reactions, where there is local lymphangitis, evidence of local necrosis at the bite site, or the rare systemic reaction, evacuate the patient. In case there is severe pain, infiltrate locally with lidocaine

For centipede bites, observe patients with minor reactions for approximately four hours, or until the reaction improves. Admit patients with evidence of significant reaction to the hospital because of potential rhabdomyolysis and acute renal failure. Tetanus prophylaxis should be current.

Note: Millipedes do not bite, but they may have secretions that irritate the skin. This can be treated by washing with soap and water (not alcohol) and applying a corticosteroid cream or lotion.

CHAPTER NINETEEN

Tick Transmitted Diseases

■ I. GENERAL INFORMATION

Several serious illnesses are transmitted by ticks to people. The most common infections are Lyme disease, Rocky Mountain spotted fever, relapsing fever, Colorado tick fever, and tick paralysis. In the Western Hemisphere, uncommon illnesses include Powassan encephalitis, babesiosis, tularemia, and ehrlichiosis.

Several measures lessen the likelihood of acquiring a tick or a tick borne illness. Clothing should be light–colored so that ticks can be more easily seen. Wear long-sleeved shirts and long pants. Tuck trousers inside a pair of high socks. Avoid contact with brush, if possible. Apply 0.5% permethrin tick repellent to clothing prior to exposure, with particular attention to the ends of shirt sleeves, pants, and collar area. A repellent containing DEET may be applied to the skin in the same areas and in other exposed locations, but overuse should be avoided, especially in children. A concentration of DEET no greater than 35% is recommended. Newer preparations containing synergists allow concentrations of less than 18% to be extremely effective. Perform a full-body inspection for ticks daily. Wash clothing after exposure.

Ticks may not attach themselves for several hours after initial skin contact and they can be easily removed. Showering or bathing may remove unattached ticks. Once they have attached themselves, removal is substantially more difficult. Because transmission of infection is frequently delayed following tick attachment, remove attached ticks immediately when discovered. If possible, preserve the tick in rubbing alcohol for later identification.

No simple, effective method is known to cause the tick to detach itself. A good method of tick removal is to gently grasp the animal with tweezers as close as possible to the point of attachment, and remove by applying gentle, direct traction. A small piece of skin may come off painlessly with the tick, which usually means that tick removal is complete. It is not always possible to remove the mouth parts with the rest of the tick. If mouth parts remain, attempt to remove them with a needle or knife point to avoid subsequent skin infection or inflammation. Avoid crushing the tick and contaminating either patient or helper with crushed tick material. Clean the wound with soap and water, and apply a bandage. Disinfect tweezers after use.

■ II. GUIDELINES FOR ASSESSMENT AND TREATMENT

A. Lyme Disease: Lyme disease is a recently recognized, widespread, tick-borne inflammatory illness caused by the *Borrelia burgdorferi* spirochete. In the United States, areas of high risk are

---

the Northeast, the upper Midwest, California, southern Oregon, and western Nevada. Most bites occur between May 1 and November 30. The first abnormality is often an expanding circular red rash (erythema chronicum migrans), which occurs around the site where the tick was attached. Flu-like symptoms often develop shortly after the rash appears.

Disseminated infection, manifested by multiple annular secondary rashes, neurologic abnormalities (meningitis, Bell's palsy, peripheral neuropathy), arthralgias, and heart involvement (most commonly AV block) may occur beginning several weeks after the tick bite.

Months after an untreated infection, arthritis may develop, usually affecting the knees and shoulders. Persistent and varied neurologic abnormalities may occur and persist for years.

Early treatment shortens the duration of erythema chronicum migrans and diminishes the likelihood of secondary and tertiary sequelae. Effective drugs at different stages of the disease are doxycycline, amoxicillin, ceftriaxone, and penicillin G.

B. Rocky Mountain Spotted Fever: In many areas of the United States (especially Montana, Oklahoma, Missouri, and the Carolinas), ticks transmit rickettsia causing Rocky Mountain spotted fever, an illness characterized initially by fever, headache, sensitivity to bright light, and muscle aches. On the third to fourth day of fever, a pink rash usually appears. If not treated promptly with antibiotics (tetracycline), the disease may be lethal.

C. Relapsing Fever: Relapsing fever is an acute febrile illness caused by *Borrelia* spirochetes. *Ornithodoros* ticks that transmit relapsing fever do not usually attach to hosts but live in the host's nest or burrow and behave more like bedbugs. Wild rodents are the intermediate hosts. Clinically, initial symptoms are those of an acute flu-like illness, but bouts continue at weekly intervals. The diagnosis is established by identification of the organism in blood smears. Tetracycline and erythromycin are effective antibiotics. Prophylactically, one should avoid rodent-infested cabins.

D. Colorado Tick Fever: This disease is an acute benign viral infection that occurs throughout the Rocky Mountain area during spring and summer. It is characterized by fever, muscle aches, and headache. The white blood cell count is usually low. The fever is often biphasic, and lasts about one week. The diagnosis is confirmed by serologic testing. There is no specific therapy.

E. Tick Paralysis: Tick paralysis begins with leg weakness. An ascending flaccid paralysis follows, which worsens as long as the tick is attached to the patient (usually a child). Speech dysfunction and difficulty swallowing are late signs, and death from aspiration or respiratory paralysis may occur. Removal of the tick results in a progressive return to normal neurologic function. Both diagnostically and therapeutically, early meticulous examination for imbedded ticks is mandatory, especially near the hairline on the neck.

■ III. CONTROVERSIES

Should prophylactic therapy be initiated following a tick bite in high-risk Lyme disease areas? Prophylactic therapy following a tick bite incurred in high risk areas is not recommended. The ticks (*Ixodes scapularis [dammini]. I. ricinus, I. pacificus*) carrying the germs that cause Lyme disease rarely transmit the infection if *attached* for less than 48 hours.

CHAPTER TWENTY

Substance Abuse in Wilderness Settings

■ I. GENERAL INFORMATION

Although data are sparse, it has been suggested that one of the single greatest contributing factors to trauma in wilderness areas is the non-prescribed and non-medically indicated use of mood- and mind-altering chemicals. Substance abuse or misuse in wilderness settings appears to be responsible for significant morbidity and mortality from acute or chronic intoxication, accidental overdoses, and withdrawal.

■ II. GUIDELINES FOR ASSESSMENT AND TREATMENT

In any individual with an illness or injury in the wilderness, mind- or mood-altering drugs may complicate assessment and treatment. Consideration must be given to whether the patient's senses are so altered as to be unaware of his or her true physical state, including the presence of pain or imminent danger. If substance abuse is suspected, take extra time to assess the patient, and give additional consideration to stabilization and care.

Working with people who are under the influence of drugs (including ethanol) is often difficult because such individuals may have radical alterations in personality, rapid mood swings, and irrational behavior patterns. A calm, unhurried, yet authoritative approach, especially with the use of a friend of the patient, can be effective in gaining the patient's confidence (or at least the patient's ear) and having him/her acquiesce to treatment.

In addition to the above, advanced providers may have two additional modalities: antidotes and sedation. Naloxone (0.4 to 4.0 mg IV, SQ), if available, will reverse the effects of narcotics and narcotic analogues. Sedation with antipsychotics (haloperidol, chlorpromazine) or with benzodiazepines (diazepam, lorazepam) can be used if patients are in danger of harming themselves or others. Extreme care must be exercised to avoid depressing the respiratory drive in such individuals.

CHAPTER TWENTY ONE

Anxiety and Stress Reactions in the Wilderness

■ I. GENERAL INFORMATION

Physical injury or accident in the back country, especially in severe cases, may be accompanied by significant psychological distress in both victim, in other party members, and even in rescuers. Panic and anxiety reactions are common in response to stressful situations. Other emotions may also occur, such as grief and depression. Victims or witnesses of traumatic injury may become so anxious that their safety (and that of other party members) is greatly compromised.

A critical incident is any situation faced by a trip participant that generates unusually strong emotional impact. These include: 1) the serious injury or death of a fellow participant 2) the serious injury or death of a bystander 3) multiple deaths or serious injuries; 4) serious injury or death of a child or infant; 5) any situation that attracts an unusual amount of attention from the media; 6) loss of life; and 7) any situation that is charged with emotion and that causes an emotional response that is beyond the normal coping mechanisms of trip members.

An immediate stress reaction is the response of a normal person to an abnormal situation, and not a sign of any psychological weakness or chronic psychiatric problems. The immediate stress reaction may include physical, emotional, cognitive, and behavioral components.

■ II. GUIDELINES FOR IMMEDIATE CARE IN THE FIELD

Medical care for physical injuries, and securing the safety of all party members, should take first priority in response to a wilderness accident. But just as one treats for shock while performing first aid or rescue operations, the psychological treatment of anxiety and stress reactions can begin almost immediately. Some basic procedures to consider in anxiety management include the following:

A. *Engage the patient in calm, rational discussion* while maintaining a focus on things that are improving (or making progress) during the first aid or rescue.

B. *Listen!* Identify the specific concerns about which the patient is anxious, and gently show that you, too, are concerned.

C. *Provide realistic/optimistic feedback.* When panic strikes, people often fear the worst and need to be brought back to objective thinking in the here-and-now.

D. *Use behavioral relaxation procedures*, especially if the patient is hyperventilating, to reduce somatic nervous system arousal; e.g., guide him or her through slow, deep breathing.

E. *Use guided imagery procedures,* such as word-pictures of pleasant events or places, to help reduce the pain.

F. *Involve the patient to the degree desired,* and to the degree possible, in actively in any decisions which must be made.

G. *Talk the patient through any technical skills* that he or she must participate in, with step-by-step advice.

■ III. MEDICATIONS

First-choice drugs for anxiety reduction are the benzodiazepines, such as diazepam (Valium®), chlordiazepoxide (Librium®), and alprazolam (Xanax®). While many drugs are effective for the symptomatic relief of anxiety (e.g., alcohol, barbiturates, and narcotic analgesics), the benzodiazepines are much safer. The primary side effect is mild sedation and, apart from potential interactions with other sedative drugs, there are very few contraindications. Therapeutic onset for anxiety relief takes from 1 to 3 hours (diazepam is the fastest acting) with typical oral dosages. Halopiridol (Haldol®) given 5 mg to 10 mg (IM or PO) is also effective in treating this disorder.

■ IV. REFERRAL AND FOLLOW-UP

Victims of traumatic events, as well as their rescuers, are at increased risk of developing post-traumatic stress disorder (PTSD); therefore, they should be educated about major symptoms that signify the need for additional treatment. Primary symptoms of PTSD include 1) distressing dreams or reliving of the trauma, 2) persistent avoidance, psychogenic amnesia, or numbing in response to trauma-related stimuli, and 3) increased somatic nervous system arousal or hyper–vigilance. Any or all of these symptoms are part of the normal human reaction to trauma, but their persistence beyond a month is diagnostic of PTSD.

Some of the most effective treatments have been developed within recent years by clinical psychologists and psychiatrists who specialize in anxiety/stress disorders. Certain cognitive-behavioral therapies and particular drugs have proven effective, alone and in various combinations. The choice of specific psychotherapeutic or pharmacologic treatment will depend on the case and type of disorder.

■ V. OTHER CONSIDERATIONS

Emotional and behavioral disorders (or psychiatric illnesses, in medical nomenclature) are common in the general adult population with incidence rates in the general adult population of 10% for anxiety disorders, 6% for major depression, and at least 5% for personality disorders. Although mountain climbers and other wilderness adventurers may be robust and seem resistant to emotional distress, some expedition members might develop psychological problems. Most people undergo emotional changes in harsh environments, and personal conflicts often add stress to group dynamics. Thus, the success of a wilderness expedition depends in part on the "people skills" of the leader or other group member.

CHAPTER TWENTY TWO

Wilderness Medical Kits

■ I. GENERAL INFORMATION

Preparations for wilderness activities include provisions for emergency care of individuals in the event of injuries or illnesses. Trip medical leaders must be able to assemble medical kits that are appropriate to support the proposed trip. This requires assessing several factors:

A. Purpose of the Trip: Selectivity is the key in choosing appropriate medical equipment. Groups intent only on providing self-treatment should consider the most common injuries they will sustain. Because a search and rescue (SAR) team must be equipped to handle the medical emergencies that they expect to encounter, they can justify carrying specialized medical gear. On recreational trips, however, the medical kit displaces other equipment that might be needed. Hikers, white water enthusiasts, and climbers all need different medical kits to meet their specialized needs.

B. Level of Medical Training: It is inappropriate to include medications and equipment that no trip member has the requisite knowledge or experience to use safely. Trip members responsible for medical care of the group should have direct input into the contents of the medical kit. Levels of training and experience can differ widely among groups of physicians, nurses, and EMS personnel. A degree or license does not guarantee knowledge in any specific area. Pre-trip training to supplement the knowledge base of the providers may be advisable.

C. Destination: The terrain, altitude, weather, propensity for endemic diseases, and other inherent dangers must be considered. Groups heading into remote areas where local inhabitants may request medical help must consider this potential demand on their supplies, and must consider whether they intend to respond.

D. Length of Trip: The total time that the party must be supported from the kit affects its contents. Some problems are likely to occur only during particular times. For example, the treatment of friction blisters is most important during the first few days of a hike. At times on a long trip, outside medical supplies can be obtained to restock the kit.

E. **Time for Evacuation or Medical Rescue:** Some trips progressively distance themselves from medical care. On other trips, time required to obtain help may be deceptive; a river raft trip into a canyon may last only hours, but evacuation in the event of an accident may take many days of dangerous and laborious effort.

F. **Size of the Party:** Although an increase in the number of participants influences the quantity of some medications and bandaging materials, the increase is not linear. Frequently, only minimal additions are needed to serve a larger group adequately. The size of the main medical kit for a large party can be reduced by equipping each member with a personal kit containing bandages, blister supplies, and personal medications.

G. **Bulk, Weight, and Cost:** Even if cost is not a consideration, the weight and bulk of a kit are potential limiting factors. Because bandaging and splints are bulky and possibly awkward to carry, the use of improvised materials, such as clothing for bandaging and local fabrication of splints, may be incorporated into plans for the medical kit. Medical equipment may also be reduced by using multi-functional components. If one piece of equipment or a drug can be used for many different purposes, weight can be significantly reduced. Knowledgeable medical team members are needed to optimize this tactic.

Some organizations and search and rescue teams use a modular approach to medical kits. Separate kits, with increasing sophistication and for various purposes, are available for individuals and situations requiring more advanced equipment. While the basic kit is designed for use by lay personnel, only specially trained individuals can use the more advanced kits, and they carry them into the field only when required.

■ II. CONTAINERS

Containers for the medical kit must be chosen for maximal accessibility and protection of contents. Damage is to be expected, and may render materials useless. In situations where there is danger of the loss of equipment, such as on white water trips, the medical kit components should be divided into several kits so that all equipment is not lost if an accident occurs. Individuals with life sustaining medications should take an extra quantity to be carried separately.

The medical kit must be easily identified and accessible when needed. This entails both making it visible, e.g. bright red and/or marked with reflective material, and placing it where it can be reached easily. Kits that unroll or open to display their contents make selection of items very convenient. For small kits, this is not usually necessary. For large kits, kits that will be used frequently, and kits that may be accessed by multiple members of the group, accessibility and easy identification of contents are very important.

■ III. GUIDELINES FOR EQUIPMENT

Equipment for a wilderness medical kit should be selected in light of its function:

A. **Life Support:** Airways, supplemental oxygen, manually-powered suction devices, chest tubes and similar equipment are generally only carried by experienced rescue personnel on prolonged remote expeditions.

B. **Vital Signs:** A watch with a second hand to time pulse or respiration is an important piece of equipment. A blood pressure cuff and stethoscope are useful in some situations, but are of no value to untrained personnel and are often considered superfluous by experienced physicians.

C. Soft Tissue Injuries: Wound closure materials range from butterfly bandages and Steri-strips®to suture equipment with surgical instruments or surgical staples. Cleansing materials, local anesthetics, and bandaging materials are also in this category. Bandaids and material for blister treatment is probably the most commonly used item in this group.

D. Orthopedic Injuries: Prefabricated splints are now manufactured in lightweight designs, including collapsible femoral traction splints, but these may be improvised in the field. Cervical collars may likewise be improvised. Backboards or litters are not usually needed, except by rescue groups. Fiberglass casting material makes an excellent light weight splinting material.

F. Medications: Special equipment in addition to the medications is necessary only if injectable drugs or intravenous fluids are carried. Injectable medications are susceptible not only to damage from bottle breakage, but also from light, heat, and cold.

■ IV. MEDICATIONS

The decision to carry any particular medication must take into account the medical knowledge required to use the medication properly, as well as the cost, bulk and weight of the kit, the potential problems that might be encountered, medication allergy history of trip participants, and knowledge of local laws and regulations that might restrict possession of certain medications.

A list of potential candidates for inclusion in this list can be obtained by referring to suggestions made in these position papers, various books on wilderness related medical care, the physician's personal medical/surgical knowledge, and standard texts and publications concerning treatment of trauma and infectious diseases. The Wilderness Medicine Letter, a publication of the Wilderness Medical Society, has run a series of articles with suggestions for customized medical kits for various remote area, climatic, and endeavor–specific activities.

CHAPTER TWENTY THREE

Immunizations

■ RESOURCES

Appropriate immunizations are vital for those entering wilderness and foreign areas. Current recommendations for U.S. travelers are issued by the Centers for Disease Control and Prevention (CDC), published annually in *Health Information for International Travel*. The publication contains vaccination and certification requirements for malaria and yellow fever on a country-by-country basis. It also includes the U.S. Public Health Service recommendations for difficult immunization questions, such as immunization of infants and pregnant or lactating women, and specific recommendations for vaccination and prophylaxis for a wide variety of disorders. It also contains a discussion of specific potential health hazards worldwide, grouped by geographic region. The information in this book is updated in the biweekly *Summary of Health Information for International Travel*. Both the book and updates can be obtained from the Superintendent of Documents, U.S. Government Printing Office, Washington, DC 20402. A weekly report of infectious diseases in the United States and important overseas medical developments is contained in the CDC publication *Morbidity and Mortality Weekly Report*. Subscriptions can be obtained from the CDC, Atlanta, GA 30333, or from the Massachusetts Medical Society, C.S.P.O. Box 9120, Waltham, MA 02254-9120, which reprints these reports as part of an inexpensive subscription service.

The Centers for Disease Control and Prevention has a hot line which provides 24 hour information on current disease status which is accessed by dialing (404) 639-1610. A FAX service is also available through this number which will return information concerning malaria prophylaxis and other disease risk factors.

The Department of State has a 24 hour hot line which provides general country information, with a travel risk assessment, at (202) 647-5225.

An alternative source of information is Vaccination Certificate Requirements and Health Advice for International Travelers, published yearly by the World Health Organization, Geneva, Switzerland. It is available through the WHO Publication Center U.S.A., 49 Sheridan Avenue, Albany, NY 12210.

The local county or state board of health will frequently have information from the above sources available for consultation and/or will have a referral service to local travel medicine specialists.

Current immunization advice, disease risk charts and other information concerning the availability of medical care within foreign countries can be obtained from IAMAT, (International Association for Medical Assistance to Travelers), 417 Center St., Lewistown, NY 14092, (716) 754-4883. IAMAT provides this information to travelers and physicians free of charge, operating only with donations.

CHAPTER TWENTY FOUR

FROM THE WILDERNESS MEDICAL SOCIETY

Wilderness Prehospital Emergency Care (WPHEC) Curriculum

Wilderness Medical Society Prehospital Committee:
E. Otten (Chairman), W. Bowman, P. Hackett, M. Spadafora, D. Tauber

Reprinted by permission of Chapman & Hall, NY.

A. Introduction

The following curriculum has been developed by the Wilderness Prehospital Emergency Care Committee of the Wilderness Medical Society (WMS) as a guide for the development and implementation of a course which is classified as a 'wilderness prehospital emergency care (WPHEC) curriculum.' *In publishing these recommendations, the WMS does not define itself as either a certifying or licensing agency.* The contents of the proposed recommendations for this curriculum represent a consensus opinion of the WMS WPHEC Committee, which is based on the personal experiences of its members, position papers on wilderness medicine published by the WMS, and study by committee members of existing courses in WPHEC. The contents of this document have been approved by the Board of Directors of the WMS. Organizations that follow these recommendations may designate their curricula as 'in accordance with the guidelines of the WMS.' This is a model curriculum; individual sections may be used based on course needs and regional circumstances. The WMS neither approves or disapproves teaching methods, nor does it test students for knowledge or skills.

Prehospital Emergency Care (PHEC) is defined as care given a patient during the time between discovery of the illness or injury and the patient's arrival at the hospital or other emergency medical facility. It can include:

(a) medical emergencies when no physician is present and the patient is in danger of imminent death;

(b) illnesses or injuries where preliminary care is necessary and appropriate to stabilize the patient, avoid further injury or complications, and allow transportation to definitive medical care; and

(c) illnesses or injuries that are not serious enough normally to require a physician's care.

Wilderness PHEC may be provided on several levels of complexity and sophistication, depending on the training of the caregivers and the amount of equipment available. The simplest level is self-help care for recreational group members, where first aid and rescue training may be at basic levels, equipment is limited, and improvisation necessary. The next higher level is Search and Rescue (SAR) group and organized Emergency Medical Services (EMS) care, where rescuers trained at least to the paramedic level may be available and equipment is more complex and sophisticated. The highest level is expeditionary emergency care given by paramedics, nurses, or physicians in isolated areas, where personnel may be highly trained and there is less emphasis on choosing equipment based on its portability.

Wilderness PHEC differs from urban PHEC in the following ways:

(1) It is provided outdoors, where the environment may be unfriendly and difficulties in obtaining food, water, and shelter may be significant. Basic survival of both the patient and caregiver may be a major concern.

(2) Definitive medical care is usually hours or days delayed, because of location, bad weather, lack of transportation, or lack of communication.

(3) Illnesses and injuries occur which are not commonly seen in the urban environment. Examples include acute mountain sickness, deep frostbite, decompression sickness, and wild animal maulings.

(4) Common illnesses and injuries require different approaches. The caregivers must learn extended care, so that complications and unnecessary disability can be prevented. the basic necessities of food, water, stabilization of body temperature, disposal of body wastes, and psychological support must be provided for each patient.

(5) Advanced medical rescue techniques, such as relocation of dislocations, wound cleansing, use of prescription drugs, intravenous fluid administration, thoracostomy tube placement, endotracheal intubation, cricothyroidotomy, and indwelling urinary catheter placement may be required.

(6) Urban protocols that rely upon rapid transport to a medical facility and radio communication with a control physician may be impossible to follow. Specially prepared wilderness protocols will be necessary.

(7) The amount of medical and first aid equipment that can be carried by a recreational wilderness party or even the best equipped wilderness SAR group with helicopter support will be limited. The caregiver must learn to improvise and choose equipment based to some extent on its weight, bulk, multiple uses, and likelihood of use.

(8) Wilderness caregivers must be realistic about their abilities to manage serious illnesses and injuries, acknowledging that fatalities will occur in circumstances where they might not if the victim could be taken rapidly to a well-equipped hospital.

(9) Certain standard urban protocols, such as the requirement that CPR be started in all cases of cardiac arrest and continued until the patient arrives at the hospital, may be unrealistic or hazardous to caregivers.

This curriculum is designed for students already trained at least to the Emergency Medical Technician—Basic level or equivalent. It will be useful as well for physicians, physicians' assistants, and nurses. These professionals often see patients after the PHEC has already been given, tend to be overly dependent on the type of medical equipment found in hospital and physicians' offices, and are not familiar with the objectives or techniques of WPHEC, either by virtue of training or experience.

In any course in WPHEC, sufficient time should be allocated to produce competence. In addition to didactic instruction, there should be ample 'hands-on' instruction, preferably conducted in an outdoor environment.

The general educational objectives of the curriculum are:

(1) To give the student a review of basic principles of anatomy, physiology, and emergency care, emphasizing their application to and, if necessary, modification for, unique problems within a wilderness environment;

(2) To give the student a review of common illnesses and injuries, emphasizing modifications of assessment and care in a wilderness environment;

(3) Instruction of the student in the causes, assessment, and treatment of *unique wilderness illnesses and injuries not typically seen in an urban environment;*

(4) Instruction of the student in *extended care* of the type needed in a wilderness environment before a victim can be evacuated to definitive medical care;

(5) Instruction of the student in the *principles of wilderness survival, SAR, and victim extrication, 'packaging,' and transportation;*

(6) To offer suggestions for contents of *wilderness emergency care kits and improvisation* of emergency equipment and supplies; and

(7) Instruction of the student in techniques of *prevention* of wilderness injuries and illnesses.

B. EMS systems

1. *Medical–legal considerations*

(a) Topics: licensing, jurisdiction, liability, duty to respond, negligence, standards of care, 'good samaritan' laws, consent, abandonment, death, coroner's case, documentation.

(b) Objective: familiarize the student with the legal environment associated with prehospital care, the importance of acting within a given scope of training, and the critical need for documentation.

2. *Communications*

(a) Topics: techniques, radio equipment and frequencies, on-line and off-line medical control, protocols.

(b) Objectives: to familiarize the student with how to set up and operate radio communication equipment, delineate the types of medical control and associated problems, and foster an understanding of the development and use of written protocols for prehospital care.

3. *Transportation*

(a) Topics: medical evacuation over ground, air, water, and ice; types of vehicles; improvisation of litters; litter and patient carries; use of pack animals; constructing and managing aircraft landing zones.

(b) Objectives: to familiarize the student with methods of transporting the sick and injured, teach how to improvise equipment, and explain the fundamentals of different types of medical evacuation.

C. First aid equipment and supplies

1. Recommended minimum

Depending on the experience and training of the individual: non-narcotic analgesics, bandages, nasal airway, splints and slings, antihistamines, epinephrine injection for allergic reactions, minor surgical instruments, laxatives, anesthetic wound infiltration, antiseptics, antibiotics, thermometer, rewarming pads and devices, snakebite kit, tourniquet, wound closure.

2. Advanced treatment modalities

Anti–arrhythmics, parenteral antibiotics, antimalarials, antidiarrheals, antivenin, narcotic analgesics, bag-valve-mask, corticosteroids, dental cement, diuretics, endotracheal tube, indwelling urinary catheter, intravenous fluids, laryngoscope, nasogastric tube, thoracostomy tube, traction splint.

D. Search and rescue (SAR) techniques

1. Organization

(a) Topics: federal, state, and local responses, National Association for Search and Rescue, planning, resources.

(b) Objectives: to teach the student how to access organizations responsible for SAR, and to plan and coordinate a SAR.

2. Operations

(a) Topics: general SAR operations, detection, patterns and techniques of search, ropes and knots, specialized equipment

(b) Objectives: to familiarize the student with the SAR operation, including personnel, equipment and supplies, and detection and search methods.

3. Unique SAR problems

(a) Topics: cave, vertical rock, mountain, surf, whitewater, lake, ice, desert, rain forest, dive, dam, flood, mineshaft, and high wind rescues.

(b) Objectives: to familiarize the student with some of the problems associated with special environmental SAR operations in order to understand the limitations of SAR personnel and equipment.

4. Environmental hazards

(a) Topics: high altitude, weather (wind, precipitation, temperature extremes, lightning), ice, avalanche, earthquake, wildfire, volcanic eruption, wild animals (dangerous, poisonous, venomous), poisonous plants and mushrooms, flood, hazardous whitewater, and ocean currents and tides.

(b) Objectives: to familiarize the student with natural environmental hazards.

E. Survival skills

1. Topics

Priorities, self rescue, personal survival kit, clothing selection, shelter and fire building, water disinfection, food gathering, signaling, celestial and compass navigation, and cold weather, desert, sea, and tropic survival.

2. Objectives

To learn the basics of survival training in diverse environments, including immediate actions necessary for basic survival, protection of a victim, planning for relocation, and acquiring additional resources.

3. Supplies

Delineation of minimum personal survival supplies and equipment.

F. Trauma management

1. Assessment

(a) Topics: mechanisms, primary survey, resuscitation, secondary survey, airway management, impalement, shock, burns, bleeding control, bandaging, splinting, recognition and treatment of infection, antitetanus immunization, pain control.

(b) Objectives: to learn the standard approach to the trauma victim based on American College of Surgeons Advanced Trauma Life Support guidelines, with enhance consideration of principles of shock prevention and treatment, care of burn wounds, basic wound care and bandaging, splinting, prevention and treatment of infection, and use of prehospital analgesics.

2. Orthopedic

(a) Topics: anatomy, fractures, dislocations, amputations, compartment syndrome, relocation, splinting, splints, slings, litter carries, improvisation.

(b) Objectives: to learn the relevant anatomy of the bones and joints, the mechanisms associated with common fractures and dislocations, and management of injuries, to include relocation,splinting, pain control, and identification of complications.

3. Neurologic

(a) Topics: anatomy, head injury, intracranial hemorrhage, concussion, increased intracranial pressure, coma, skull fracture, seizure, spinal cord injury, cervical spine immobilization, and central and peripheral neurologic exam.

(b) Objectives: to learn the basic anatomy of the brain and spinal cord, identification of common injuries, a method for a pertinent and simplied neurologic exam, and treatment of head injuries, spinal cord injuries, increased intracranial pressure, and spinal cord injuries.

4. Eye, ear, nose, and throat

(a) Topics: anatomy, occluded airway, eye protection, ocular foreign body, corneal abrasion, eye infections, snow blindness, eye patching, intraocular injuries, epistaxis, facial fractures, tooth avulsion, toothache, mandible dislocation, laryngeal injury, ear infections, sinus infections, pharyngitis, and perforated tympanic membrane.

(b) Objectives: to learn the basic anatomy of the eyes, ears, nose and throat; common eye injuries and the proper technique for patching an eye; control of epistaxis, reduction of a dislocated mandible; and identification and remediation of life-threatening airway problems.

5. Chest

(a) Topics: anatomy, pneumothorax, tension, pneumothorax, rib fractures, flail chest, pulmonary contusion, sucking chest wound, pericardial tamponade, heart and great vessel injury, tracheal injury, esophageal foreign body, and needle and tube thoracostomy.

(b) Objectives: to learn the basic anatomy of the thorax and its contents; identification of common injuries; and treatment for manageable intrathoracic injuries.

6. Abdomen/pelvis

(a) Topics: anatomy, intra-abdominal injuries, pelvic fractures, straddle injuries, urinary retention, use of military anti-shock garment.

(b) Objectives: to learn the basic anatomy of the abdomen and pelvis; identification of intra-abdominal injury; treatment for evisceration of abdominal contents, urinary retention, and pelvic and genital injuries.

7. Special trauma

(a) Topics: the pregnant victim, the pediatric victim, blast injuries, gunshot wounds, barotrauma, asphyxiation, avalanche injuries.

(b) Objectives: to learn the unique problems associated with trauma during pregnancy; the injured child; and the mechanisms involved in ballistic injuries, blast injuries, underwater injuries, and the specific types of injuries encountered in avalanche and landslide victims.

G. Medical Emergencies

1. Cardiorespiratory

(a) Topics: cardiac arrests, myocardial ischemia and infarction, chest pain, pulmonary edema, asthma.

(b) Objectives: to learn basic cardiorespiratory physiology; identification of the patient with cardiac arrest, pulmonary edema, myocardial infarction or ischemia, and the specific therapeutic modalities for each; evaluation and management of the patient with chest pain; guidelines for initiation, continuation, and discontinuation of CPR in the setting of a wilderness environment; evaluation and treatment of the patient with asthma or other reactive airway disease.

2. Gastrointestinal

(a) Topics: abdominal pain, the acute abdomen, gastrointestinal hemorrhage, nausea and vomiting, diarrhea, constipation, hemorrhoids.

(b) Objectives: to learn the basic anatomy and physiology of the gastrointestinal tract; signs and symptoms of the common causes of abdominal pain; the acute abdomen; appropriate therapeutic modalities; the evaluation and management of gastrointestinal hemorrhage, nausea, vomiting and diarrhea; fluid and electrolyte replacement; prevention and treatment of hemorrhoids and constipation.

3. Genitourinary

(a) Topics: renal colic, urinary tract infection, vaginal and pelvic infection, vaginal bleeding, pregnancy, and childbirth.

(b) Objectives: to learn the basic anatomy and physiology of the genitourinary system; evaluation and management of the patient with kidney stones; vaginal hemorrhage and conditions related to pregnancy; emergency childbirth and problems unique to the wilderness environment.

4. Metabolic/allergic

(a) Topics: diabetes, hypoglycemia, ketoacidosis, allergic reactions, anaphylaxis.

(b) Objectives: to learn the immediate and long-term management of problems related to diabetes; evaluation, management and prevention of local systemic allergic reactions and anaphylaxis.

5. Neurologic
(a) Topics: headache, cerebrovascular accidents, seizures.
(b) Objectives: to learn the basic anatomy and physiology of the nervous system; evaluation and management of the patient with headache, seizures, and cerebrovascular accident.

6. Infectious disease
(a) Topics: upper respiratory tract infections, pneumonia, urinary tract infections, gastroenteritis, infectious diarrhea, cutaneous infections, otologic and odontogenic infections, hepatitis, immunizations.
(b) Objectives: to learn evaluation and management of the patient with upper respiratory tract, head, and neck infections, such as pharyngitis, otitis, bronchitis, sinusitis, and dental abscess; evaluation and management of the patient with pneumonia; signs and symptoms of gastroenteritis and infectious diarrhea, including treatment principles and preventive techniques; recognition and treatment of superficial and deep cutaneous infections; evaluation and management of genitourinary tract infections; signs and symptoms of hepatitis; immunization principles for foreign travel.

H. Environmental emergencies
1. Physical
(a) Topics: high altitude physiology, high altitude pulmonary edema, high altitude cerebral edema, acute mountain sickness, hypothermia, cold water immersion, frostbite, near-drowning, lightning injury, heat illness, sunburn.
(b) Objectives: to learn the physiological changes that occur at altitude; understand the signs and symptoms of altitude illnesses, and their prevention and treatment; the body's response to heat and cold; the signs and symptoms of hypothermia, frostbite, heat cramps, heat exhaustion, and heat stroke; prevention and treatment of disorders related to environmental temperature; treatment of near-drowning and lightning injuries; the effects of ultraviolet radiation on the skin and eyes; prevention and treatment of solar radiation-induced injuries.

2. Plants
(a) Topics: poisonous plants, poisonous mushrooms, plant dermatitis.
(b) Objectives: to become familiar with common poisonous plants and mushrooms; signs, symptoms, and treatment of poisoning; principles of therapy regarding contact dermatitis.

3. Animals
(a) Topics: venomous marine animals, arthropods, and snakes; nonvenomous animal bites and injuries; rabies; tick-borne diseases; mosquito-borne diseases; other zoonoses.
(b) Objectives: to become familiar with the common venomous animals and insects of North America, including animal identification, signs and symptoms of envenomation, and treatment modalities for bites and stings; care for nonvenomous bite wounds, recognition and treatment of common zoonoses.

I. Psychological emergencies

(a) Topics: acute psychosis, patient restraint, drug abuse, grief, depression, stress management.

(b) Objectives: to learn the presentations of common psychological problems, including grief response, acute psychosis, post-traumatic stress disorder, and depression; problems associated with drug abuse; methods of patient restraint.

J. Disaster planning and triage

(a) Topics: natural disasters, mass casualties, triage, resources, planning.

(b) Objectives: to study various types of disasters, the types of casualties encountered, principles of triage, and the organization of an immediate response.

K. Preventive medicine

(a) Topics: international travel, immunizations, malaria prophylaxis, diarrhea prevention, physical conditioning.

(b) Objectives: to learn unique medical problems associated with travel to foreign countries, the role of and requirements for immunizations; the physical conditioning as a means of prevention of illnesses and injuries.

The Scope of Wilderness Medicine

Our interests include the following areas:

- Physiologic interactions of environmental forces on human performance and health

- Environmental health disorders
    Heat illness
    Hypothermia, hyperthermia
    Frostbite
    Altitude illness
    Barotrauma submersion

- Health risks in specific environments
    Mountains
    Deserts
    Jungles
    Marine
    Aerospace
    Subterranean (caves)

- Health risks from plants and animals
    Toxinology
    Animal attacks

- Traditional medicine in remote environments
    Wilderness trauma
    Medical limitations to wilderness travel

- Travel medicine

- Medical services in wilderness settings
    Search and rescue
    Organization of wilderness medical services
    Expedition medicine

- Infectious diseases from the wilderness and foreign travel

- Liability in wilderness medicine

- Education in wilderness medicine

- Global health issues from environmental depredation

Share our Members' Sense of Adventure

Our physician and professional members are committed to expanding their knowledge of the prevention, diagnosis and treatment of wilderness diseases and injuries.

Society members include experts in high–altitude physiology and medical problems from exposure to heat and cold. Others work with astronauts and aquanauts or treat the victims of animal attacks, poisonous bites and stings. Many WMS members play an integral role in wilderness medical issues within government, civic and medical organizations.

Mission Statement

The purpose of the Wilderness Medical Society is to encourage, foster, support or conduct activities or programs concerned with life sciences that can improve the scientific knowledge of the membership and the general public in matters related to wilderness environments and human activities in these environments.

The mission of the Wilderness Medical Society is to establish an organization composed of qualified physicians, allied health specialists and other qualified individuals that will concern itself with matters related to wilderness medicine and the benefits, health, safety and medical care of the individual in the wilderness.

Dear Wilderness Medicine Enthusiast,

This is your special invitation to join the Wilderness Medical Society, the largest organization in the world devoted to wilderness medical issues. The Society is traditional in its commitment to medical knowledge, education and research. Yet, it is unique in its focus on wilderness environments and the challenges they present.

As a Society member, you will join physicians and other professionals who share medical, conservation and recreational interest in wilderness activities. You will have a wealth of opportunities and materials for professional and personal growth such as clinical journals, publications, slide–lecture sets and accredited scientific meetings. In addition, you will have ample opportunity to play a leadership role in the Society.

Regular membership in the Wilderness Medical Society is an outstanding value at only $90 per year, which includes your journal subscription. Whether you are an accomplished wilderness traveler and an expert in wilderness medicine or you are just beginning to cultivate your interest in the field, the Wilderness Medical Society is for you.

We look forward to your favorable reply.

Cordially,

The Board of Directors
Wilderness Medical Society

Membership Application

Please complete the form below and mail it along with the dues for the appropriate membership category to: The Wilderness Medical Society, P.O. Box 2462, Indianapolis, IN 46206.

NAME _____ DATE _____

ADDRESS _____

CITY _____

STATE _____ ZIP _____

TELEPHONE HOME _____

BUSINESS _____ FAX _____

Sponsoring member (if applicable) _____

My primary interest in the Wilderness Medical Society is: _____
_____

How did you find out about the Wilderness Medical Society? _____
_____

Medical specialty, if any _____

_____ Regular member—$90/year, (includes journal subscription)
_____ Associate/Student member—$30/year
_____ Associate/Student member with journal subscription—$80/year
_____ Corporate member—$1,000/year

M/C OR VISA NO. _____

EXPIRATION DATE _____ SIGNATURE _____

WILDERNESS MEDICAL SOCIETY
P O Box 2463, Indianapolis, IN 46204
Phone: 317.631.1745 Fax: 317.269.8150

SCHEDULE OF EDUCATIONAL CONFERENCES

Fifth Annual Winter Wilderness Medicine Conference
March 6–11, 1995
Keystone Resort
Keystone, Colorado

Second World Congress on Wilderness Medicine
August 8–12, 1995
The Ritz–Carlton
Aspen, Colorado

Desert and Tropical Medicine Conference
October 11–15, 1995
Sheraton El Conquistador
Tucson, Arizona

Sixth Annual Winter Wilderness Medicine Conference
February 10–16, 1996
Big Sky Resort
Big Sky, Montana

Travel and Environmental Medicine Conference
April 24–28, 1996
Sweeney Convention Center
Santa Fe, New Mexico

11th Annual Scientific Meeting
August 3–9, 1996
The Lodge at Kananaskis
Kananaskis, Alberta, Canada

Seventh Annual Winter Wilderness Medicine Conference
February 1–7, 1997
Sheraton Steamboat Resort
Steamboat Springs, Colorado

Diving and Marine Medicine Conference
1997
Date & Location TBA

12th Annual Scientific Meeting
August 2–8, 1997
Sun Valley Resort
Sun Valley, Idaho

Eighth Annual Winter Wilderness Medical Conference
February 14–21, 1998
Snowbird Ski and Summer Resort
Snowbird, Utah